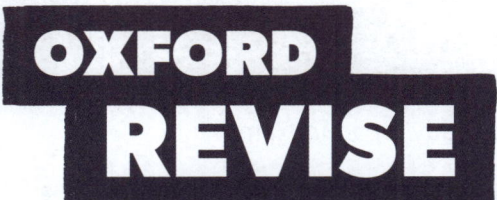

AQA GCSE HISTORY

Britain: Health and the people: c1000 to the present day

COMPLETE REVISION AND PRACTICE

Series Editor: Aaron Wilkes
Harriet Power
Aaron Wilkes

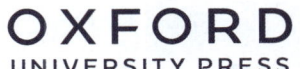

Contents

 Shade in each level of the circle as you feel more confident and ready for your exam.

How to use this book — iv

Part one: Medicine stands still — 2-11

Part two: The beginnings of change — 12-21

1 Medieval medicine and medical progress — 2
 Knowledge
 Retrieval
 Practice

3 The impact of the Renaissance on Britain — 12
 Knowledge
 Retrieval
 Practice

2 Public health in the Middle Ages — 8
 Knowledge
 Retrieval
 Practice

4 Dealing with, and preventing, disease — 16
 Knowledge
 Retrieval
 Practice

FACTORS

You need to know the importance of the following factors in the history of medicine. Look out for the following icons as you work through each Knowledge Organiser.

 Religion   Technology and Science

 War   Chance

 Individual   Communication

 Government

You can use the following mnemonic to help you remember the factors: **R**on **W**easley **I**s **G**inger: **T**hat's **S**o **Ch**uffin' **C**ool!

REVISION TIP

Your study ranges across a thousand years of history and you need to compare aspects of medicine across the periods studied, so make sure you understand your chronology. You will see BCE, meaning 'Before the Common Era', in relation to Ancient Greece and Rome. CE starts after 0BCE.

Part one covers the later medieval period (c1000–c1500); Part two covers the Renaissance and Enlightenment (c1500–c1800); Part three covers the Industrial Revolution (c1800–c1900); and Part four covers the modern period (c1900+). You will need to link themes and factors across these periods.

ii

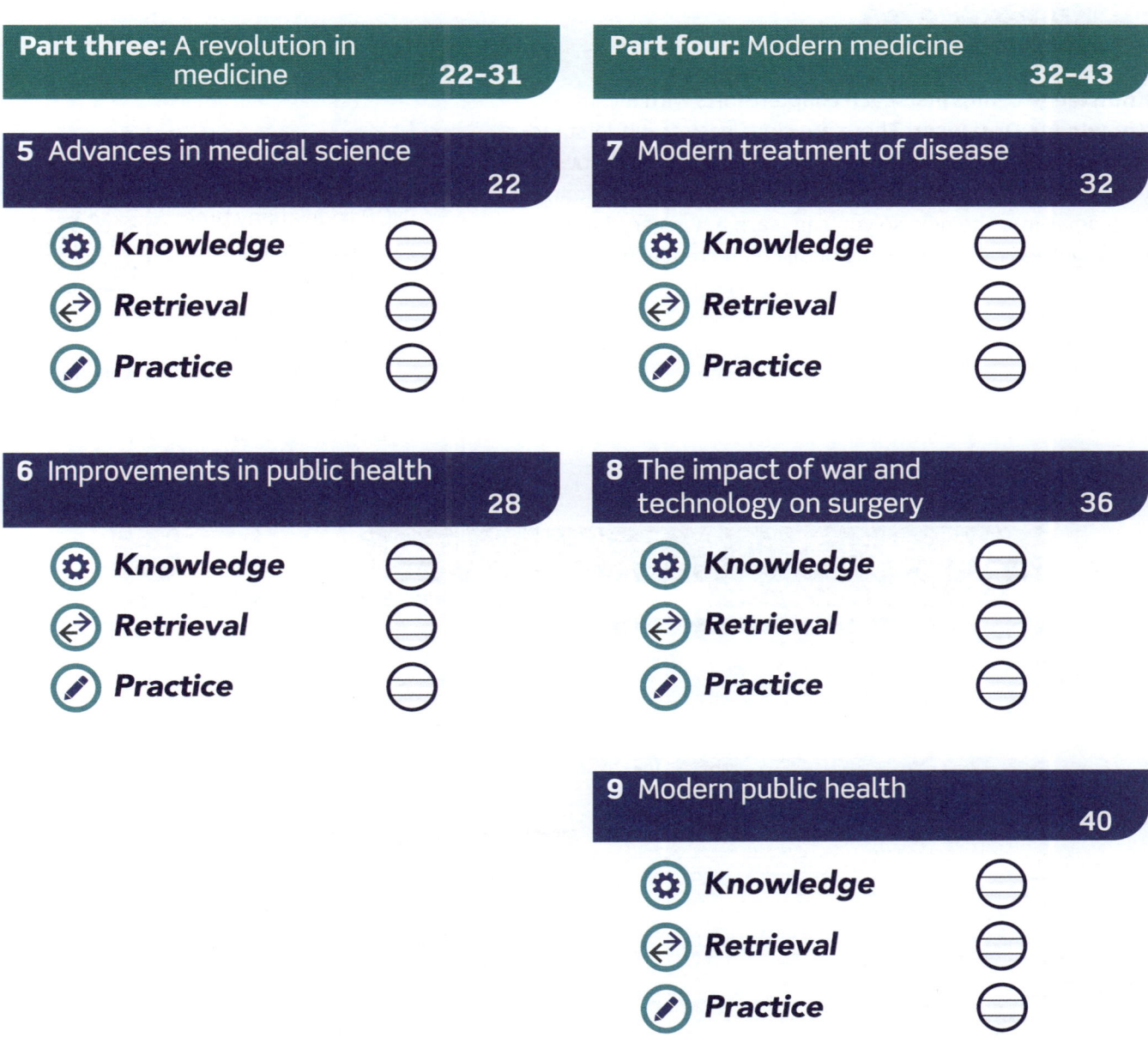

Part three: A revolution in medicine 22-31

5 Advances in medical science 22
- Knowledge
- Retrieval
- Practice

6 Improvements in public health 28
- Knowledge
- Retrieval
- Practice

Part four: Modern medicine 32-43

7 Modern treatment of disease 32
- Knowledge
- Retrieval
- Practice

8 The impact of war and technology on surgery 36
- Knowledge
- Retrieval
- Practice

9 Modern public health 40
- Knowledge
- Retrieval
- Practice

How to use this book

This book uses a three-step approach to revision: **Knowledge**, **Retrieval**, and **Practice**. It is important that you do all three; they work together to make your revision effective.

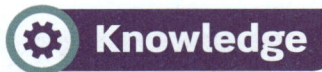

Knowledge

Knowledge comes first. Each chapter starts with a **Knowledge Organiser**. These are clear, easy-to-understand, concise summaries of the content that you need to know for your exam. The information is organised to show how one idea flows into the next so you can learn how everything is tied together, rather than lots of disconnected facts.

Answers and Glossary

You can scan the QR code at any time to access sample answers mark schemes for all the exam-style questions, a glossary containing definitions of the key terms, as well as further revision support. go.oup.com/OR/GCSE/A/Hist/Health

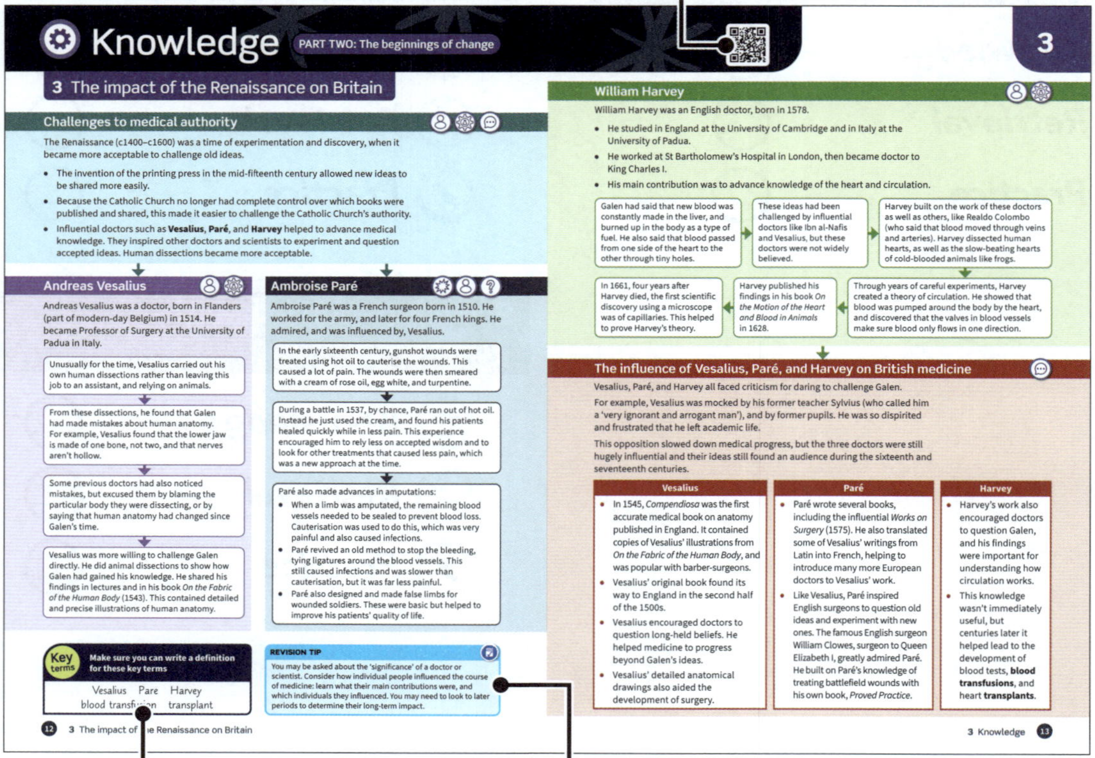

Knowledge PART TWO: The beginnings of change

3 The impact of the Renaissance on Britain

Challenges to medical authority

The Renaissance (c1400–c1600) was a time of experimentation and discovery, when it became more acceptable to challenge old ideas.

- The invention of the printing press in the mid-fifteenth century allowed new ideas to be shared more easily.
- Because the Catholic Church no longer had complete control over which books were published and shared, this made it easier to challenge the Catholic Church's authority.
- Influential doctors such as **Vesalius**, **Paré**, and **Harvey** helped to advance medical knowledge. They inspired other doctors and scientists to experiment and question accepted ideas. Human dissections became more acceptable.

Andreas Vesalius

Andreas Vesalius was a doctor, born in Flanders (part of modern-day Belgium) in 1514. He became Professor of Surgery at the University of Padua in Italy.

Unusually for the time, Vesalius carried out his own human dissections rather than leaving this job to an assistant, and relying on animals.

From these dissections, he found that Galen had made mistakes about human anatomy. For example, Vesalius found that the lower jaw is made of one bone, not two, and that nerves aren't hollow.

Some previous doctors had also noticed mistakes, but excused them by blaming the particular body they were dissecting, or by saying that human anatomy had changed since Galen's time.

Vesalius was more willing to challenge Galen directly. He did animal dissections to show how Galen had gained his knowledge. He shared his findings in lectures and in his book *On the Fabric of the Human Body* (1543). This contained detailed and precise illustrations of human anatomy.

Ambroise Paré

Ambroise Paré was a French surgeon born in 1510. He worked for the army, and later for four French kings. He admired, and was influenced by, Vesalius.

In the early sixteenth century, gunshot wounds were treated using hot oil to cauterise the wounds. This caused a lot of pain. The wounds were then smeared with a cream of rose oil, egg white, and turpentine.

During a battle in 1537, by chance, Paré ran out of hot oil. Instead he just used the cream, and found his patients healed quickly while in less pain. This experience encouraged him to rely less on accepted wisdom and to look for other treatments that caused less pain, which was a new approach at the time.

Paré also made advances in amputations:

- When a limb was amputated, the remaining blood vessels needed to be sealed to prevent blood loss. Cauterisation was used to do this, which was very painful and also caused infections.
- Paré revived an old method to stop the bleeding, tying ligatures around the blood vessels. This still caused infections and was slower than cauterisation, but it was far less painful.
- Paré also designed and made false limbs for wounded soldiers. These were basic but helped to improve his patients' quality of life.

Key terms — Make sure you can write a definition for these key terms

Vesalius Pare Harvey blood transfusion transplant

REVISION TIP

You may be asked about the 'significance' of a doctor or scientist. Consider how individual people influenced the course of medicine: learn what their main contributions were, and which individuals they influenced. You may need to look to later periods to determine their long-term impact.

12 3 The impact of the Renaissance on Britain

3

William Harvey

William Harvey was an English doctor, born in 1578.

- He studied in England at the University of Cambridge and in Italy at the University of Padua.
- He worked at St Bartholomew's Hospital in London, then became doctor to King Charles I.
- His main contribution was to advance knowledge of the heart and circulation.

Galen had said that new blood was constantly made in the liver, and burned up in the body as a type of fuel. He also said that blood passed from one side of the heart to the other through tiny holes.

These ideas had been challenged by influential doctors like Ibn al-Nafis and Vesalius, but these doctors were not widely believed.

Harvey built on the work of these doctors as well as others, like Realdo Colombo (who said that blood moved through veins and arteries). Harvey dissected human hearts, as well as the slow-beating hearts of cold-blooded animals like frogs.

Through years of careful experiments, Harvey created a theory of circulation. He showed that blood was pumped around the body by the heart, and discovered that the valves in blood vessels make sure blood only flows in one direction.

Harvey published his findings in his book *On the Motion of the Heart and Blood in Animals* in 1628.

In 1661, four years after Harvey died, the first scientific discovery using a microscope was of capillaries. This helped to prove Harvey's theory.

The influence of Vesalius, Paré, and Harvey on British medicine

Vesalius, Paré, and Harvey all faced criticism for daring to challenge Galen.

For example, Vesalius was mocked by his former teacher Sylvius (who called him a 'very ignorant and arrogant man'), and by former pupils. He was so dispirited and frustrated that he left academic life.

This opposition slowed down medical progress, but the three doctors were still hugely influential and their ideas still found an audience during the sixteenth and seventeenth centuries.

Vesalius	Paré	Harvey
• In 1545, *Compendiosa* was the first accurate medical book on anatomy published in England. It contained copies of Vesalius' illustrations from *On the Fabric of the Human Body*, and was popular with barber-surgeons. • Vesalius' original book found its way to England in the second half of the 1500s. • Vesalius encouraged doctors to question long-held beliefs. He helped medicine to progress beyond Galen's ideas. • Vesalius' detailed anatomical drawings also aided the development of surgery.	• Paré wrote several books, including the influential *Works on Surgery* (1575). He also translated some of Vesalius' writings from Latin into French, helping to introduce many more European doctors to Vesalius' work. • Like Vesalius, Paré inspired English surgeons to question old ideas and experiment with new ones. The famous English surgeon William Clowes, surgeon to Queen Elizabeth I, greatly admired Paré. He built on Paré's knowledge of treating battlefield wounds with his own book, *Proved Practice*.	• Harvey's work also encouraged doctors to question Galen, and his findings were important for understanding how circulation works. • This knowledge wasn't immediately useful, but centuries later it helped lead to the development of blood tests, **blood transfusions**, and heart **transplants**.

3 Knowledge 13

Key terms — Make sure you can write a definition for these key terms

The **Key terms** box highlights the key words and phrases you need to know, remember, and be able to use confidently.

REVISION TIP

Revision tips offer you helpful advice and guidance to aid your revision and help you to understand key concepts and remember them.

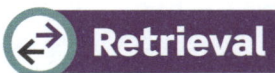

Retrieval

The **Retrieval questions** help you learn and quickly recall the information you've acquired. These are short questions and answers about the content in the Knowledge Organiser you have just reviewed. Cover up the answers with some paper and write down as many answers as you can from memory. Check back to the Knowledge Organiser for any you got wrong, then cover the answers and attempt all the questions again until you can answer *all* the questions correctly.

Make sure you revisit the Retrieval questions on different days to help them stick in your memory. You need to write down the answers each time, or say them out loud, otherwise it won't work.

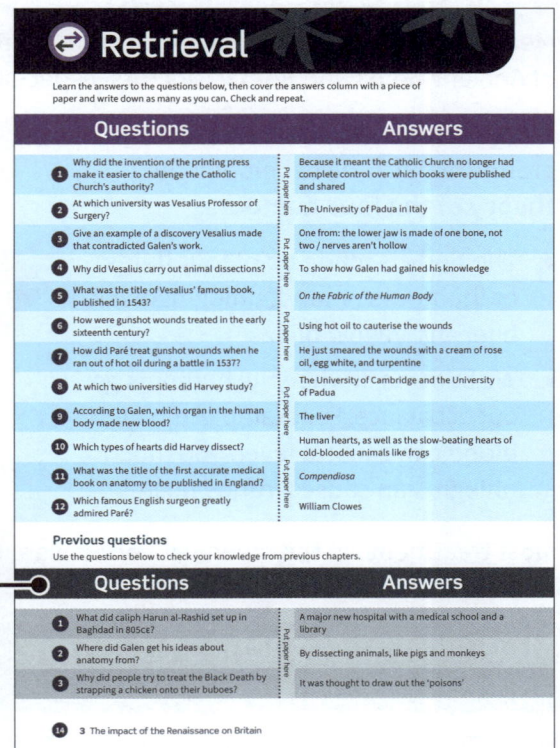

Previous questions

Each chapter also has some **Retrieval questions** from **previous chapters**. Answer these to see if you can remember the content from the earlier chapters. If you get the answers wrong, go back and do the Retrieval questions for the earlier chapters again.

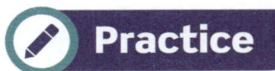

Practice

Once you think you know the Knowledge Organiser and Retrieval answers really well, you can move on to the final stage: **Practice**.

Each chapter has **exam-style questions**, including some questions from previous chapters, to help you apply all the knowledge you have learnt and can retrieve.

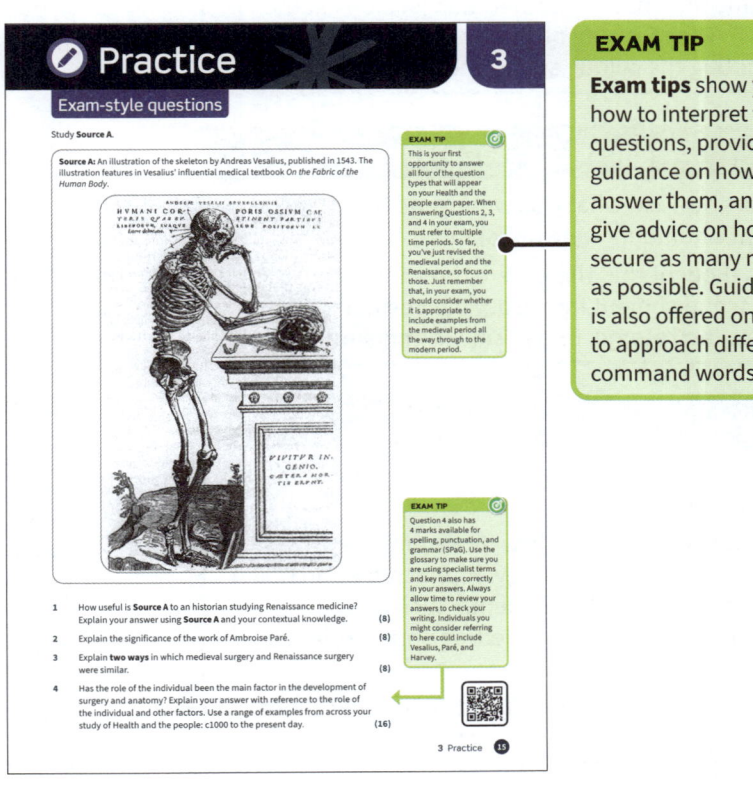

EXAM TIP

Exam tips show you how to interpret the questions, provide guidance on how to answer them, and give advice on how to secure as many marks as possible. Guidance is also offered on how to approach different command words.

v

 # Knowledge

PART ONE: Medicine stands still

1 Medieval medicine and medical progress

The ideas of Hippocrates and Galen

Medicine in late medieval England (c1000–c1500) was strongly influenced by the writings of Ancient Greek and Roman doctors, especially **Hippocrates** and **Galen**.

Hippocrates was a Greek doctor born around 460BCE. He developed the **theory of the four humours**:

- The body is made up of four fluids or 'humours': blood, phlegm, black bile, and yellow bile.
- We become ill when the humours get out of balance. For example, too much blood can cause a fever. Too much phlegm can cause a runny nose.

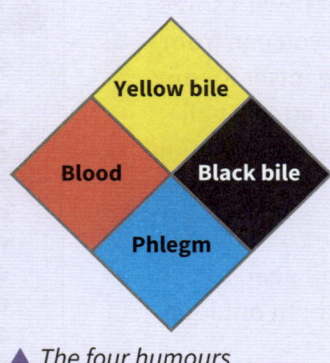

▲ *The four humours*

Galen was a Greek doctor born in 129CE. He built on Hippocrates' work to develop the **theory of opposites**:

- Illness can be cured by balancing the humours.
- For example, if a person has too much blood, they should be treated with **bloodletting**. If they have too little blood, they should drink red wine or eat red meat.

Most treatments in the medieval period were based on the theory of opposites.

Medieval approaches to diagnosis and treatment

Doctors in medieval England needed to observe and diagnose their patients before deciding how to treat them.

1 Observation

Hippocrates' teaching encouraged doctors to examine their patient (rather than just look at the illness). They focused on taking the patient's pulse and noting the colour, smell, and taste of their urine.

2 Diagnosis (causes of illness)

Doctors decided what was wrong and how the patient's humours were unbalanced.

It was thought that there were three main causes of illness: punishment from God, the position of the planets (**astrology**), or bad smells (**miasma**).

3 Treatment

Doctors aimed to restore the balance of the humours with treatment.

Supernatural treatments were common, such as prayers, charms or astrology. Hippocrates and Galen encouraged **natural** treatments, such as herbs and certain foods, or bloodletting and **purging**, to balance the humours.

Ultimately, people believed that God would choose whether to cure someone or not.

Medieval doctors and other healers

The best person to visit when ill in medieval England was a doctor (also known as a **physician**).

- Doctors' training involved studying medicine at a university for at least seven years.
- They mainly learned by attending lectures and reading books, rather than interacting with patients.
- Their knowledge was taken from Ancient Greece and Rome – particularly Hippocrates and Galen – and combined with Islamic, Chinese, and Indian ideas.

There weren't many trained doctors, however, and most people weren't wealthy enough to afford them. Instead, ill people sought help from:

- a local wise person: these healers used a mixture of herbal remedies, first aid, and supernatural cures. Much of their knowledge was passed down by word of mouth, from one generation to the next
- a **barber-surgeon**, who performed small surgical procedures like bloodletting and extracting teeth
- a local monastery or parish priest: many medieval hospitals were based in religious buildings and provided free care
- an **apothecary**, who sold herbs and spices.

The contribution of Christianity to medical progress

Christianity was the main religion in medieval Europe and the Christian Church influenced the study and practice of medicine.

The Christian Church taught that it was important to look after the sick like Jesus did, and that illness was a punishment or a test of faith from God.

Christians believed that God decided whether someone would recover from their illness. This meant treatments often focused on trying to please God and asking God for help. They included praying to God, donating to the Church, and going on **pilgrimage** to shrines.

How Christianity helped medicine

- ✅ The Church respected the traditional medical knowledge of the Ancient Greeks and Romans. Monks preserved and studied this knowledge.
- ✅ The Church controlled the training of doctors in universities.
- ✅ The Church thought doctors should give spiritual comfort, for example by explaining why God might make a person ill. This helped patients to die in peace.
- ✅ The Church provided free care.

How Christianity held back medicine

- ❌ The Church approved of Galen because he believed in a single God, as Christians do. This made it difficult for anyone to challenge Galen's incorrect ideas, as this would be seen as going against the Church.
- ❌ The Church discouraged doctors from exploring new ideas.
- ❌ The Church disproved of human **dissections**, making it harder for doctors to learn about human **anatomy**.
- ❌ The Church did not think doctors should heal people. Hospitals were for comfort only.

Medieval hospitals

Between c1000 and c1500, more than 700 hospitals were started in England.

Common features of medieval hospitals

- Many were financed by the Church. Some were supported by a wealthy patron (a sponsor or supporter).
- Often based in religious buildings such as monasteries.
- Many were small, with room for only 12 patients (the number of Jesus' disciples). Some were larger: one of the largest in England was St Leonard's in York, which could look after 200 people.
- Many were quiet, clean places where people could rest. These hospitals focused more on caring for patients than curing them. They provided food and prayers.
- Many did not have doctors and did not provide medical treatment. Instead they were run by monks or nuns, with a priest providing spiritual support.
- Many did not just take in people who were ill. They also looked after orphans, the elderly, and those experiencing poverty.
- Many did not take in patients who were **contagious** (or who were thought to be contagious). Specialist hospitals were set up for these patients instead. For example, 'Lazar houses' were set up outside towns for people with leprosy (a contagious disease that affects the skin and nerves).

Mental illness was considered contagious, so separate hospitals for the mentally ill were set up, such as Bedlam in London.

Key terms

Make sure you can write a definition for these key terms

Hippocrates   Galen   theory of the four humours
theory of opposites   bloodletting   astrology   miasma
supernatural   natural   purging   physician
barber-surgeon   apothecary   pilgrimage
dissection   anatomy   contagious   amputation   cauterisation
anaesthetic   trepanning   antiseptic   ligature

Knowledge — PART ONE: Medicine stands still

1 Medieval medicine and medical progress

Islamic medicine and surgery

By 750CE, the large Islamic Empire stretched across northern Africa and the Middle East. This empire was ruled by a series of caliphs.

During the medieval period, Islamic medicine was more advanced than medicine in Western Europe.

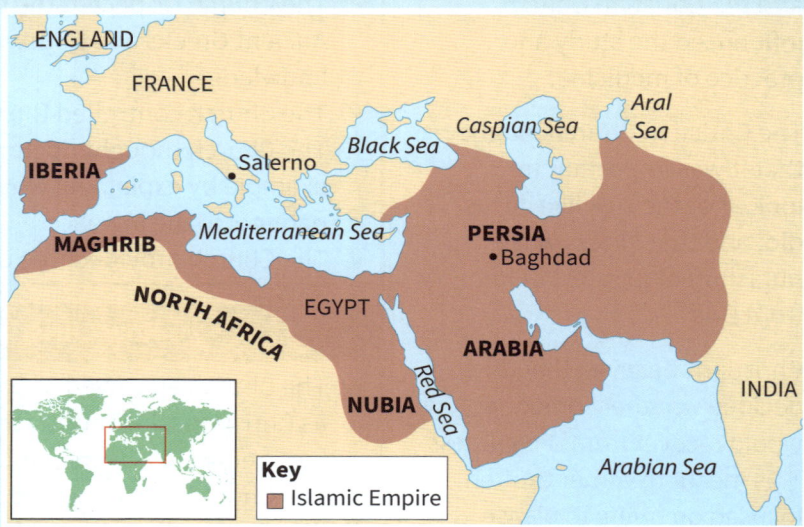

▶ The Islamic Empire, c750CE

Reasons why Islamic medicine progressed in the medieval period

Support from the caliphs
- Many caliphs were interested in science and supported the development of medicine. For example, caliph Harun al-Rashid set up a new hospital in Baghdad in 805CE, with a medical school and a library.
- Al-Rashid also encouraged Greek medical books to be translated into Arabic, and built up a large library. His son, caliph al-Mamun, developed the library into the world's largest at the time, and a study centre for scholars.

Support from Islam
- Islam encouraged medical learning. Islamic hospitals actively tried to cure patients (rather than simply care for them), and doctors were usually present.
- Prophet Muhammad (the founder of Islam) inspired people to 'seek learning even as far as China' and said that, for every disease, God has given a cure. Doctors and scientists were encouraged to seek out these cures.

Challenging Galen
- In Western Europe, the Catholic Church discouraged people from challenging Galen's ideas. In the Islamic Empire, people had more freedom to challenge traditional views about medicine.
- The famous doctor Al-Razi (known in Europe as Rhazes) believed, like Galen, that it was important to observe patients carefully and use natural (rather than supernatural) treatments. However, he also criticised some of Galen's ideas: one of his books was called *Doubts About Galen*.
- Another well-known doctor, Ibn Sina (known in Europe as Avicenna), used observation and testing to build on Galen's views. He discovered new causes of pain, and improved Galen's theory of how the pulse works.

The importance of Islamic medicine

✓ Pioneering Islamic doctors and scientists wrote books about their discoveries. Some of these books were translated into Latin and introduced into Western Europe.

For example, Ibn Sina's book, *Canon of Medicine*, was translated into Latin in the twelfth century. This encyclopaedia became the standard medical textbook used to teach doctors in Western Europe until the seventeenth century.

✗ Not all ideas made it across to Western Europe. For example, the Muslim doctor Ibn al-Nafis was the first to describe how blood circulated around the body via the lungs. This challenged Galen's idea that blood passed straight from the right-hand side of the heart to the left-hand side. But al-Nafis' books weren't read in Western Europe and Galen's mistake was accepted in Western Europe until the seventeenth century.

Surgery in medieval times

- Medieval surgery was risky and painful, and often only used as a last resort. The dangers of blood loss, shock, and infection led to low rates of survival.
- Medieval understanding of anatomy was limited. Many ideas about the body were based on Galen's dissection of animals, like pigs and monkeys. Even when human dissections became more accepted in the fourteenth century, and it became clearer that some of Galen's ideas about anatomy were wrong, it was still unpopular to challenge his views.
- Most surgery took place on battlefields, in wars such as the Crusades and the Hundred Years' War.

The main medieval surgical procedures included the following.

Technique	What it involved
Bloodletting	- Making a small cut on the inside of the arm, to let the blood run out - Thought to restore the balance of the humours in the body
Amputation	- Cutting off a painful or damaged part of the body
Cauterisation	- Burning a wound to stop it bleeding, usually by heating a piece of iron and pressing it onto the wound - Would stop the bleeding, but was immensely painful and often infected the wound
Anaesthetics	- Putting a patient to sleep or numbing the pain of surgery by giving them natural substances like mandrake root, hemlock, or opium - Not used very often as too strong a dose could kill a patient; instead, patients were held down during surgery
Trepanning	- Drilling a hole in a person's skull. This was thought to allow demons to escape, which would 'cure' conditions like epilepsy - Most people died, but some survived the procedure

Medieval surgeons

Barber-surgeons performed most of the surgery in the medieval period. They learned what to do by being apprenticed to another surgeon, or by learning on the battlefield.

Some surgeons experimented with new methods, and shared their ideas through writing. Pioneering surgeons included:

Hugh of Lucca and his son Theodoric

- Italian surgeons who criticised the common view (based on the theory of opposites) that pus was needed for a wound to heal.
- Instead of encouraging wounds to create pus, they closed the wounds up quickly and then used wine as an **antiseptic** to reduce the chances of infection.
- However, their ideas did not catch on as they were challenged by the influential French surgeon Guy de Chauliac, who criticised their work in his textbook *Great Surgery* (1363). This textbook dominated English and French surgical knowledge for 200 years.

John of Arderne

- An English surgeon who combined Greek and Arab knowledge with his experience of serving in the Hundred Years' War.
- His book *Practica* (1376) included illustrations of his operations and instruments.
- He was renowned for developing a safer treatment for anal abscesses (swellings that were common among knights who spent a lot of time on horseback).

Al-Zahrawi

- A Muslim surgeon known in Europe as Abulcasis.
- He wrote *Al Tasrif*, an encyclopaedia of medical practices, in 1000CE.
- He invented 26 new surgical instruments.
- He pioneered using **ligatures** to tie off blood vessels and using catgut for internal stitches.
- He made cauterisation popular.

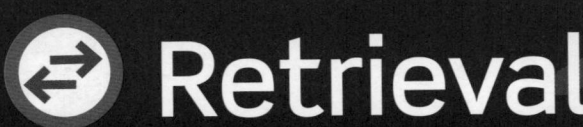

Retrieval

Learn the answers to the questions below, then cover the answers column with a piece of paper and write down as many as you can. Check and repeat.

Questions | Answers

#	Question	Answer
1	Who developed the theory of the four humours?	Hippocrates
2	Name the four humours.	Blood, phlegm, black bile, and yellow bile
3	Who developed the theory of opposites?	Galen
4	When examining patients, what did medieval doctors focus on?	Taking the patient's pulse and noting the colour, smell, and taste of their urine
5	What were considered to be the three main causes of illness in medieval England?	Punishment from God, the position of the planets (astrology), and bad smells (miasma)
6	Are charms and astrology considered supernatural or natural treatments?	Supernatural
7	What did training involve for medieval doctors?	Studying medicine at a university for at least seven years; attending lectures and reading books
8	In medieval England, how did wise people learn their medical knowledge?	Much of their knowledge was passed down by word of mouth, from one generation to the next
9	What was the main religion in medieval Europe?	Christianity
10	Where were hospitals in medieval England often based?	In religious buildings such as monasteries
11	What were 'Lazar houses'?	Specialist hospitals for people with leprosy
12	What did caliph Harun al-Rashid set up in Baghdad in 805CE?	A new hospital with a medical school and a library
13	Which book from the Islamic Empire became the standard medical textbook used to teach doctors in Western Europe until the seventeenth century?	*Canon of Medicine* by Ibn Sina (Avicenna)
14	Where did Galen get his ideas about anatomy from?	By dissecting animals, like pigs and monkeys
15	What did cauterisation involve in the medieval period?	Burning a wound to stop it bleeding, usually by heating a piece of iron and pressing it onto the wound
16	What did trepanning involve in the medieval period?	Drilling a hole in a person's skull to allow demons to escape
17	Which two Italian surgeons criticised the view that pus was needed for a wound to heal?	Hugh of Lucca and his son Theodoric
18	Which medieval surgeon made cauterisation popular?	Al-Zahrawi (known as Abulcasis in Europe)

1 Medieval medicine and medical progress

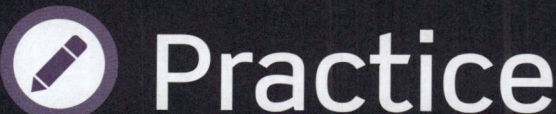# Practice

Exam-style questions

There will be **four** questions on your Health and the people exam paper. However, Questions 2, 3, and 4 all require you to think about more than one time period, so we'll wait until Chapter 3 to introduce them, when you'll have revised the medieval period and the Renaissance.

> **EXAM TIP**
>
> Before attempting to answer each question, use the 'BUG' method:
> - **Box the command word**, so that you know what you are being asked to do.
> - **Underline the key words** (the words that tell you which topic the question is about, and jog your memory about the topic).
> - **Glance at the question again**, to pick up any additional information it is giving you and to help you picture what you need to do.

Study **Source A**.

Source A: A French illustration, from c1500. The illustration shows the Hotel Dieu hospital in Paris, which was a large hospital run by the Catholic Church.

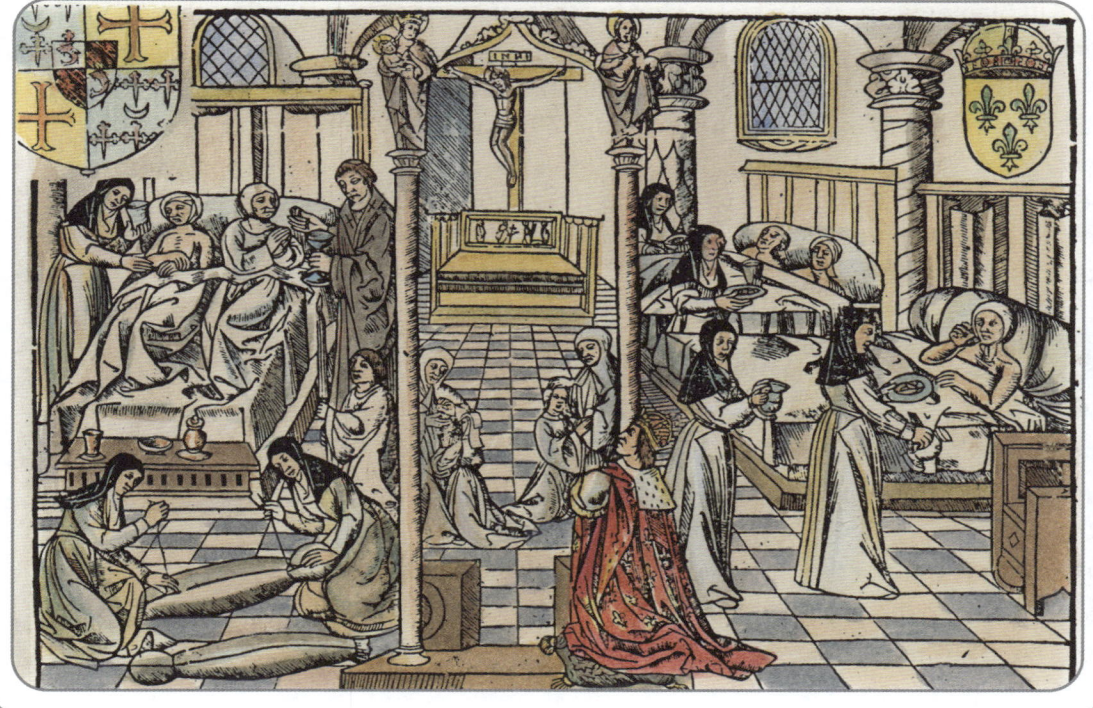

1 How useful is **Source A** to an historian studying medieval medicine? Explain your answer using **Source A** and your contextual knowledge. **(8)**

> **SOURCE TIP**
>
> Look carefully at the source. What does it show about how patients are cared for? Who is looking after patients? What does it show about the setting? Compare this to your own knowledge of medieval hospitals: does it match what you know was common for the time?

> **SOURCE TIP**
>
> When analysing a source, you need to consider not just its content but also its provenance (who it is by, when and where it was published, what type of artwork it is, its title, and so on). Read the caption to the source carefully, as this will give you information about its provenance. For example, for this source, you might think about the date the illustration was created, and the type of hospital it shows.

Knowledge

PART ONE: Medicine stands still

2 Public health in the Middle Ages

Towns and cities

In English towns and cities in the **Middle Ages**, **public health** was generally poor. A main reason for this was how waste was handled.

Waste from toilets	Waste from businesses
• Some people used a bucket as a toilet and threw the waste onto the street. • Most towns (and some wealthy individuals) built **privies** with **cesspits** underneath to collect the waste. The cesspits were emptied by **gong farmers**, who were meant to take the waste outside the town walls, but sometimes dumped it in a nearby river. • When the cesspits overflowed in heavy rain, sewage spilled out into the streets.	• Businesses usually dumped their waste either directly into the river or in open drains that ran down the middle of streets, which washed waste into a nearby river when it rained. • Some waste products were unhygienic or dangerous, such as blood and guts from butchers, or deadly chemicals from leather tanners.

However, there were some attempts to improve conditions. For example:
- In 1330, the council in Glamorgan passed a law to stop butchers throwing animal remains into the high street.
- In 1374, a London council introduced a fee for households who dumped their sewage in the Walbrook stream. The council used the money to have the stream cleaned each year.
- In 1388, Parliament passed a law that meant people who threw 'dung, garbage, and entrails' into ditches, ponds, and rivers could be fined £20. (This law was hard to enforce and many people ignored it.)

> **REVISION TIP**
> Learning specific examples helps you add depth to your answers and support your arguments. For example, memorise one or two of the laws introduced to improve public health in the Middle Ages.

Monasteries

Monasteries were often situated in isolated places, but close to a river. This source of flowing water was important for maintaining good health conditions:
- Elaborate systems of pipes delivered water from the river to the **lavatorium**, where monks washed themselves.
- Filtering systems removed impurities by allowing dirt to settle out of the water.
- Waste water was emptied into the river.
- Toilets and cesspits were flushed out occasionally by diverting the river water through them.

There were also other reasons why monasteries tended to be more hygienic, healthier places than medieval towns and cities:

Reasons why monasteries had good health conditions:
- Monasteries were very wealthy. This meant monks had enough money to build good **sanitation** facilities.
- Isolation helped to protect them from infectious **epidemics**.
- Cleanliness was encouraged because it was considered a sign of piety (being devoted to your religion).
- Monks lived simple, disciplined lives with a balanced diet (and good sleep and exercise) to balance the humours.
- Monks were educated and had access to medical books in their libraries. They knew about the basic principles of good sanitation, such as keeping clean water and waste water separate.

What was the Black Death?

The Black Death was a deadly **pandemic** that started in Asia and quickly spread to Western Europe. It reached England in 1348, and the rest of Britain in 1349.

- Historians believe the Black Death was a combination of two diseases: **bubonic plague** and **pneumonic plague**.
- The Black Death killed nearly half of Europe's population, and at least 1.5 million people in Britain. Victims developed swellings (buboes) filled with pus.

Causes of the Black Death

At the time, no one understood how the Black Death spread. It was blamed on things such as God being angry, the position of the stars and planets, or bad air. Historians now believe it was mainly caused by the **bacteria** *Yersinia pestis*.

Black rats carried *Yersinia pestis* in their blood. The rats probably brought the Black Death to England by travelling on ships from Asia. 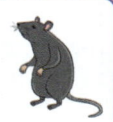	Fleas living on the rats bit them and they became infected. 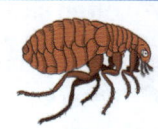
If the plague reached their lungs, the person could spread it through the air by coughing or sneezing. This pneumonic plague was even more deadly. 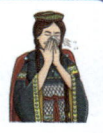	When a rat died, its fleas looked for a new host. If the fleas jumped onto a person and bit them, the person became infected and developed bubonic plague. 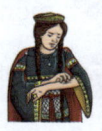

Prevention and treatment

At the time, no one knew how to prevent or treat the Black Death. It spread quickly because:

- people lived close together in crowded towns and cities
- the pneumonic form of the plague easily spread through the air
- bodies were disposed of badly, sometimes in shallow pits that wild animals dug up at night
- the filth and waste that littered streets gave rats the perfect environment to breed and increase in number.

Treatment	Prevention
- People tried all sorts of treatments, from drinking mercury and bloodletting to strapping a chicken onto their buboes. This was thought to draw out the 'poisons'. - In some European countries, people used **flagellation** to ask for forgiveness from God. - There was no cure that actually worked.	- Many people realised they could catch the Black Death from others. They tried to avoid contact with people who were obviously ill. - Some people carried **pomanders** to ward off the bad smells thought to cause the Black Death. - In some European countries (particularly Italy), **quarantines** were introduced in some towns. For example, in Venice in Italy, ships had to wait for 40 days before people were allowed to come ashore. - In England, some local councils tried to quarantine travellers or people with symptoms, but this wasn't widespread or well enforced.

Key terms — Make sure you can write a definition for these key terms

Middle Ages   public health   privy   cesspit   gong farmer   lavatorium   sanitation   epidemic   pandemic   bubonic plague   pneumonic plague   bacteria   flagellation   pomander   quarantine

Retrieval

Learn the answers to the questions below, then cover the answers column with a piece of paper and write down as many as you can. Check and repeat.

Questions / Answers

#	Question	Answer
1	What were gong farmers meant to do with the waste from cesspits?	Take it outside the town walls
2	What did businesses in medieval towns and cities usually do with their waste?	Dump it either directly into the river or in open drains that ran down the middle of streets
3	In 1330, how did the council in Glamorgan try to improve the cleanliness of this region's towns and cities?	It passed a law to stop butchers throwing animal remains into the high street
4	Where were monasteries in the Middle Ages often situated?	In isolated places, close to a river
5	How did monasteries clean out their toilets and cesspits?	By occasionally diverting the river water through them to flush them out
6	Why was cleanliness encouraged in medieval monasteries?	Because it was considered a sign of piety
7	In which year did the Black Death reach England?	1348
8	Name the two diseases that historians believe made up the Black Death.	Bubonic plague and pneumonic plague
9	How many people died in Britain from the Black Death?	At least 1.5 million
10	One way the Black Death spread was through infected people coughing and sneezing. What was the other way?	Fleas that were infected with *Yersinia pestis* biting people
11	Why did people try to treat the Black Death by strapping a chicken onto their buboes?	It was thought to draw out the 'poisons'
12	What did some people carry to ward off the bad smells thought to cause the Black Death?	Pomanders

Previous questions

Use the questions below to check your knowledge from previous chapters.

#	Question	Answer
1	Name the four humours.	Blood, phlegm, black bile, and yellow bile
2	Where were hospitals in medieval England often based?	In religious buildings such as monasteries
3	What did cauterisation involve in the medieval period?	Burning a wound to stop it bleeding, usually by heating a piece of iron and pressing it onto the wound

2 Public health in the Middle Ages

Practice

Exam-style questions

There will be **four** questions on your Health and the people exam paper. However, Questions 2, 3, and 4 all require you to think about more than one time period, so we'll wait until Chapter 3 to introduce them, when you'll have revised the medieval period and the Renaissance.

Study **Source A**.

Source A: An English engraving of the Black Death from 1348. The engraving shows a plague sufferer covered in what may be pustules (pus-filled blisters). Some medieval scholars noted that this was a common symptom. The lightning and flames in the background are symbolic of the destruction caused by the plague.

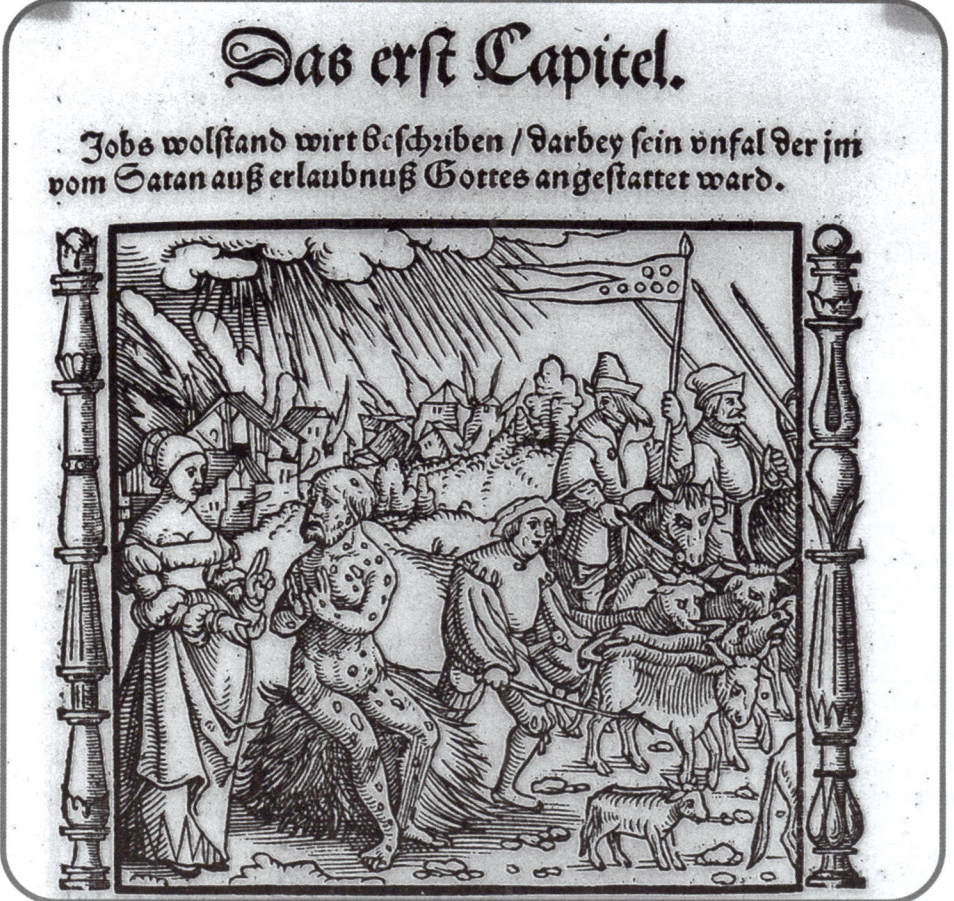

> **SOURCE TIP**
>
> Consider when the source was created and what it shows about the effects of the plague (both on individuals and on society as a whole).

> **SOURCE TIP**
>
> Use your own knowledge of the Black Death to help you answer this question. For example, the provenance tells you that this engraving was created in England in 1348. Why is that year significant, and why does it mean this engraving is useful to an historian studying the Black Death?

1. How useful is **Source A** to a historian studying the Black Death? Explain your answer using **Source A** and your contextual knowledge. **(8)**

Knowledge

PART TWO: The beginnings of change

3 The impact of the Renaissance on Britain

Challenges to medical authority

The Renaissance (c1400–c1600) was a time of experimentation and discovery, when it became more acceptable to challenge old ideas.

- The invention of the printing press in the mid-fifteenth century allowed new ideas to be shared more easily.
- Because the Catholic Church no longer had complete control over which books were published and shared, this made it easier to challenge the Catholic Church's authority.
- Influential doctors such as **Vesalius**, **Paré**, and **Harvey** helped to advance medical knowledge. They inspired other doctors and scientists to experiment and question accepted ideas. Human dissections became more acceptable.

Andreas Vesalius

Andreas Vesalius was a doctor, born in Flanders (part of modern-day Belgium) in 1514. He became Professor of Surgery at the University of Padua in Italy.

> Unusually for the time, Vesalius carried out his own human dissections rather than leaving this job to an assistant, and relying on animals.

> From these dissections, he found that Galen had made mistakes about human anatomy. For example, Vesalius found that the lower jaw is made of one bone, not two, and that nerves aren't hollow.

> Some previous doctors had also noticed mistakes, but excused them by blaming the particular body they were dissecting, or by saying that human anatomy had changed since Galen's time.

> Vesalius was more willing to challenge Galen directly. He did animal dissections to show how Galen had gained his knowledge. He shared his findings in lectures and in his book *On the Fabric of the Human Body* (1543). This contained detailed and precise illustrations of human anatomy.

Ambroise Paré

Ambroise Paré was a French surgeon born in 1510. He worked for the army, and later for four French kings. He admired, and was influenced by, Vesalius.

> In the early sixteenth century, gunshot wounds were treated using hot oil to cauterise the wounds. This caused a lot of pain. The wounds were then smeared with a cream of rose oil, egg white, and turpentine.

> During a battle in 1537, by chance, Paré ran out of hot oil. Instead he just used the cream, and found his patients healed quickly while in less pain. This experience encouraged him to rely less on accepted wisdom and to look for other treatments that caused less pain, which was a new approach at the time.

> Paré also made advances in amputations:
> - When a limb was amputated, the remaining blood vessels needed to be sealed to prevent blood loss. Cauterisation was used to do this, which was very painful and also caused infections.
> - Paré revived an old method to stop the bleeding, tying ligatures around the blood vessels. This still caused infections and was slower than cauterisation, but it was far less painful.
> - Paré also designed and made false limbs for wounded soldiers. These were basic but helped to improve his patients' quality of life.

Key terms — Make sure you can write a definition for these key terms

Vesalius   Paré   Harvey   blood transfusion   transplant

REVISION TIP

You may be asked about the 'significance' of a doctor or scientist. Consider how individual people influenced the course of medicine: learn what their main contributions were, and which individuals they influenced. You may need to look to later periods to determine their long-term impact.

William Harvey

William Harvey was an English doctor, born in 1578.

- He studied in England at the University of Cambridge and in Italy at the University of Padua.
- He worked at St Bartholomew's Hospital in London, then became doctor to King Charles I.
- His main contribution was to advance knowledge of the heart and circulation.

Galen had said that new blood was constantly made in the liver, and burned up in the body as a type of fuel. He also said that blood passed from one side of the heart to the other through tiny holes.

→ These ideas had been challenged by influential doctors like Ibn al-Nafis and Vesalius, but these doctors were not widely believed.

→ Harvey built on the work of these doctors as well as others, like Realdo Colombo (who said that blood moved through veins and arteries). Harvey dissected human hearts, as well as the slow-beating hearts of cold-blooded animals like frogs.

↓

In 1661, four years after Harvey died, the first scientific discovery using a microscope was of capillaries. This helped to prove Harvey's theory.

← Harvey published his findings in his book *On the Motion of the Heart and Blood in Animals* in 1628.

← Through years of careful experiments, Harvey created a theory of circulation. He showed that blood was pumped around the body by the heart, and discovered that the valves in blood vessels make sure blood only flows in one direction.

↓

The influence of Vesalius, Paré, and Harvey on British medicine

Vesalius, Paré, and Harvey all faced criticism for daring to challenge Galen.

For example, Vesalius was mocked by his former teacher Sylvius (who called him a 'very ignorant and arrogant man'), and by former pupils. He was so dispirited and frustrated that he left academic life.

This opposition slowed down medical progress, but the three doctors were still hugely influential and their ideas still found an audience during the sixteenth and seventeenth centuries.

Vesalius

- In 1545, *Compendiosa* was the first accurate medical book on anatomy published in England. It contained copies of Vesalius' illustrations from *On the Fabric of the Human Body*, and was popular with barber-surgeons.
- Vesalius' original book found its way to England in the second half of the 1500s.
- Vesalius encouraged doctors to question long-held beliefs. He helped medicine to progress beyond Galen's ideas.
- Vesalius' detailed anatomical drawings also aided the development of surgery.

Paré

- Paré wrote several books, including the influential *Works on Surgery* (1575). He also translated some of Vesalius' writings from Latin into French, helping to introduce many more European doctors to Vesalius' work.
- Like Vesalius, Paré inspired English surgeons to question old ideas and experiment with new ones. The famous English surgeon William Clowes, surgeon to Queen Elizabeth I, greatly admired Paré. He built on Paré's knowledge of treating battlefield wounds with his own book, *Proved Practice*.

Harvey

- Harvey's work also encouraged doctors to question Galen, and his findings were important for understanding how circulation works.
- This knowledge wasn't immediately useful, but centuries later it helped lead to the development of blood tests, **blood transfusions**, and heart **transplants**.

Retrieval

Learn the answers to the questions below, then cover the answers column with a piece of paper and write down as many as you can. Check and repeat.

Questions | Answers

#	Question	Answer
1	Why did the invention of the printing press make it easier to challenge the Catholic Church's authority?	Because it meant the Catholic Church no longer had complete control over which books were published and shared
2	At which university was Vesalius Professor of Surgery?	The University of Padua in Italy
3	Give an example of a discovery Vesalius made that contradicted Galen's work.	One from: the lower jaw is made of one bone, not two / nerves aren't hollow
4	Why did Vesalius carry out animal dissections?	To show how Galen had gained his knowledge
5	What was the title of Vesalius' famous book, published in 1543?	*On the Fabric of the Human Body*
6	How were gunshot wounds treated in the early sixteenth century?	Using hot oil to cauterise the wounds
7	How did Paré treat gunshot wounds when he ran out of hot oil during a battle in 1537?	He just smeared the wounds with a cream of rose oil, egg white, and turpentine
8	At which two universities did Harvey study?	The University of Cambridge and the University of Padua
9	According to Galen, which organ in the human body made new blood?	The liver
10	Which types of hearts did Harvey dissect?	Human hearts, as well as the slow-beating hearts of cold-blooded animals like frogs
11	What was the title of the first accurate medical book on anatomy to be published in England?	*Compendiosa*
12	Which famous English surgeon greatly admired Paré?	William Clowes

Previous questions

Use the questions below to check your knowledge from previous chapters.

Questions | Answers

#	Question	Answer
1	What did caliph Harun al-Rashid set up in Baghdad in 805CE?	A major new hospital with a medical school and a library
2	Where did Galen get his ideas about anatomy from?	By dissecting animals, like pigs and monkeys
3	Why did people try to treat the Black Death by strapping a chicken onto their buboes?	It was thought to draw out the 'poisons'

3 The impact of the Renaissance on Britain

Practice

Exam-style questions

Study **Source A**.

Source A: An illustration of the skeleton by Andreas Vesalius, published in 1543. The illustration features in Vesalius' influential medical textbook *On the Fabric of the Human Body*.

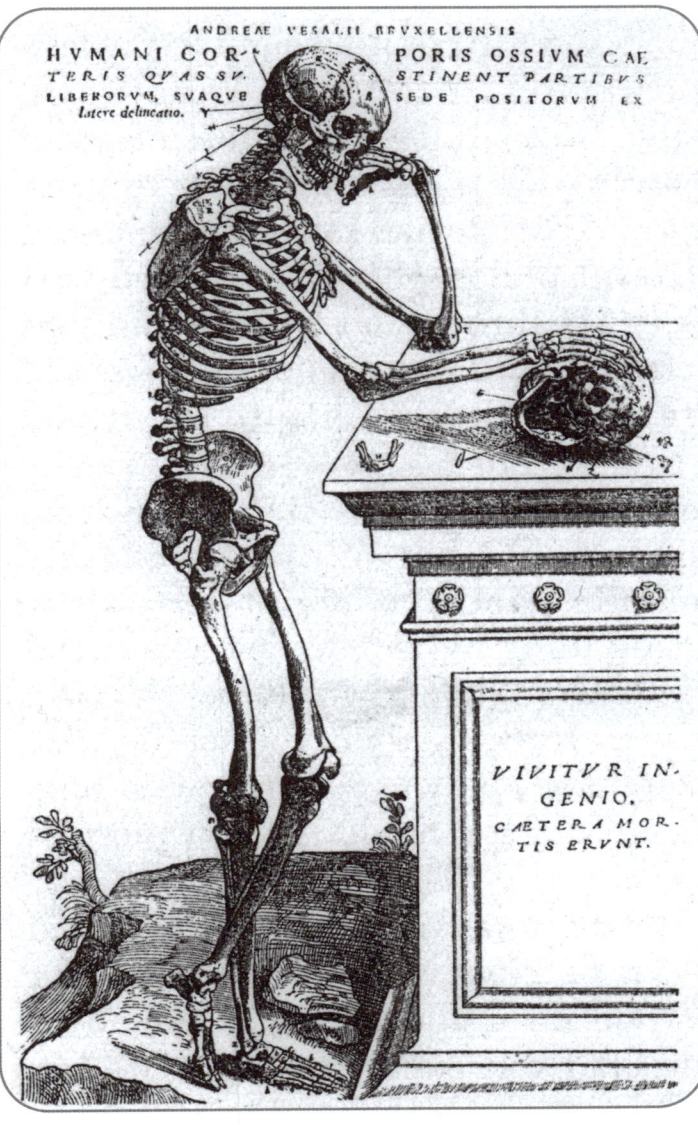

> **EXAM TIP**
>
> This is your first opportunity to answer all four of the question types that will appear on your Health and the people exam paper. When answering Questions 2, 3, and 4 in your exam, you must refer to multiple time periods. So far, you've just revised the medieval period and the Renaissance, so focus on those. Just remember that, in your exam, you should consider whether it is appropriate to include examples from the medieval period all the way through to the modern period.

> **EXAM TIP**
>
> Question 4 also has 4 marks available for spelling, punctuation, and grammar (SPaG). Use the glossary to make sure you are using specialist terms and key names correctly in your answers. Always allow time to review your answers to check your writing. Individuals you might consider referring to here could include Vesalius, Paré, and Harvey.

1. How useful is **Source A** to an historian studying Renaissance medicine? Explain your answer using **Source A** and your contextual knowledge. (8)

2. Explain the significance of the work of Ambroise Paré. (8)

3. Explain **two ways** in which medieval surgery and Renaissance surgery were similar. (8)

4. Has the role of the individual been the main factor in the development of surgery and anatomy? Explain your answer with reference to the role of the individual and other factors. Use a range of examples from across your study of Health and the people: c1000 to the present day. (16)

Knowledge — PART TWO: The beginnings of change

4 Dealing with, and preventing, disease

Seventeenth- and eighteenth-century medicine

The Renaissance encouraged a more scientific and questioning approach to medicine among some (such as Vesalius and Paré) in the sixteenth century, but many doctors still relied on traditional treatments and ideas in the seventeenth and eighteenth centuries.

Traditional treatments and ideas	New treatments and ideas
• Treatments were still based on the four humours, such as bloodletting and purging. • Surgical techniques such as cauterisation were still used. Surgery remained dangerous and painful. • Most people couldn't afford to see a trained doctor. Instead, they relied on barber-surgeons for minor operations, and apothecaries and wise people for herbal remedies. • Apothecaries and wise people still relied on traditional knowledge that had been passed down through generations. (Some of their remedies did work, such as using willow bark to dull pain.) • Many people still held superstitious beliefs, such as the idea that the king's touch could cure scrofula.	• The invention of the printing press made it easier to share books on medicine. For example, the English doctor Nicholas Culpeper published *The Complete Herbal* in 1653, to share his understanding of herbal remedies. • Explorers brought back new natural medicines from other countries. For example, opium from Turkey began to be used as an anaesthetic and cinchona bark from South America was used to treat malaria. • Inspired by Vesalius and others who questioned Galen, some doctors experimented with new ideas. • In 1677, the use of microscopes allowed scientists to discover microorganisms.

Quackery

Quacks were showy salespeople who pretended to have medical knowledge. They were popular in the seventeenth and eighteenth centuries.

- Quacks travelled from town to town, selling 'miracle' cures. One such cure was Daffy's Elixir: an 'elixir of health' that was said to cure anything.
- The medicines sold by quacks usually did nothing to help people recover, but they were popular because:

| They were cheap compared to paying for a doctor. | They were expertly marketed at a time when there were few effective cures for illness. | They often contained enough alcohol or opium to mask a person's symptoms for long enough to convince them the medicine was working. |

Some doctors were critical of quacks and favoured a scientific approach rooted in observation and practical experience. Thomas Sydenham was one such doctor.

Sydenham advocated taking a restrained approach (letting the body heal itself) rather than purging and bloodletting. He introduced effective treatments, such as laudanum for pain relief and iron for anaemia.

Key terms — Make sure you can write a definition for these key terms: quack, Great Plague, social distancing, dispensary, Hunter, placebo, Jenner, inoculation, vaccination

The Great Plague

The Black Death returned to Britain a number of times. In 1665, it killed around 100,000 people in London and thousands more in the rest of the country. This outbreak is known as the **Great Plague**.

Similarities to the Black Death	Differences to the Black Death
<ul><li>People were still unaware of the real cause of the disease: infected fleas living on rats. They still thought the plague was caused by God, the position of the planets, or bad air.</li><li>There was still no cure. Ineffective treatments still included, for example, bloodletting and using animals to 'draw out the poison'.</li><li>People still used pomanders to ward off bad smells.</li></ul>	There was a more organised approach to dealing with the plague that made use of quarantines and **social distancing**:<ul><li>The British government quarantined all ships coming into London.</li><li>'Searchers', who were usually knowledgeable local women, were paid to identify people suffering from the plague. These people were then quarantined in their houses, which were identified with a red cross on the door. Watchmen made sure they didn't leave.</li><li>In 1666, King Charles II banned all public gatherings (such as plays and funerals).</li><li>There was also a growing understanding that dirt and filth were connected to disease. For example, people were ordered to sweep the streets in front of their houses.</li><li>The bodies of those who had died were brought out at night (when fewer people were about), then buried in mass pits.</li></ul>

The growth of hospitals

- Medieval hospitals were often small and funded by the Catholic Church. When King Henry VIII turned against the Catholic Church in the 1530s, many monasteries (and their hospitals) were shut down.
- New hospitals needed to be built in their place. These were funded in various ways: by the monarch, by businesses, charities or wealthy individuals, or by 'private subscription' (local people coming together to jointly pay for the hospital).
- In 1700, there were two general hospitals in London. Five new general hospitals were added between 1720 and 1750, and nine more throughout the rest of Britain. By 1800, London's hospitals cared for over 20,000 patients a year.

Eighteenth-century hospitals were similar in some ways to medieval hospitals, but there were also improvements.

> **REVISION TIP**
> You may get an exam question asking you about the similarities between medicine in different periods in history. Try to remember these similarities as you revise.

Similarities to medieval hospitals	Differences to medieval hospitals
<ul><li>Treatments were still based on the four humours, with a reliance on bloodletting and purging.</li><li>Surgery was still only carried out as a last resort, due to how dangerous and painful it was.</li><li>Hospitals still provided free care to people living in poverty.</li><li>Doctors were still unaware of the importance of cleanliness for preventing disease.</li><li>There were some specialist hospitals, such as St Luke's Hospital for the mentally ill (opened 1751) and the Foundling Hospital for children (opened 1741).</li></ul>	<ul><li>Hospitals became places to try to treat patients, not just care and pray for them.</li><li>Doctors and nurses now looked after patients, rather than monks and nuns.</li><li>The new hospitals were built to care for hundreds of patients. Specialist wards were set up, dedicated to particular diseases or procedures.</li><li>Medical schools were often attached to the new hospitals. They helped to given student doctors more hands-on experience.</li><li>**Dispensaries** were added to hospitals towards the end of the eighteenth century. They gave out medicines for free.</li></ul>

Knowledge

PART TWO: The beginnings of change

4 Dealing with, and preventing, disease

The training and status of surgeons and physicians

Surgeons were less respected than physicians in the seventeenth century, but they gained more respect and their training became more formalised during the eighteenth century.

Physicians	Surgeons
• Physicians had the highest status in medicine, and were thought to provide the best care. • They were doctors who had studied medicine at university. • They specialised in diagnosing patients and prescribing medicines or treatments; they rarely performed surgery themselves. • They were expensive and mostly treated wealthy people or royalty as a result.	• Surgery was painful, dangerous, and limited in what it could achieve. • Surgeons and barber-surgeons were seen as craftsmen, and not as respected as physicians. • Rather than studying at university, they usually trained through an apprenticeship: learning from another surgeon (sometimes on the battlefield). • During the eighteenth century, surgery slowly became more valued as it advanced and became more scientific. Surgeons grew in status. • This led to the Company of Surgeons splitting away from the Company of Barber-Surgeons in 1745. The new company established a base near Newgate jail, so it could teach trainee surgeons by dissecting executed criminals. • Surgeons started to learn by studying at the medical schools attached to hospitals.

John Hunter

John **Hunter** was a Scottish surgeon, born in 1728.

- He worked as an army surgeon, set up his own practice in London, and became King George III's surgeon.
- He was a keen researcher who aimed to use a scientific approach of experimentation and careful observation.
- For example, Hunter observed that mercury appeared to be an ineffective treatment for gonorrhoea. He set up an experiment where he gave some patients mercury pills and others bread pills (as a **placebo**). He found that all the patients got better, regardless of which pills they took.
- Similar to Paré, Hunter took a restrained approach to healing gunshot wounds. He disagreed with the common practice of cutting out the area around a gunshot wound because it was thought to be poisonous.
- He also refrained from carrying out amputations on wounded soldiers unless it was absolutely necessary.
- Hunter wrote several books and trained hundreds of other surgeons (including Edward **Jenner**) in his scientific approach.
- He was interested in anatomy and built up a huge collection of human and animal body parts. He encouraged other surgeons to study anatomy to gain a better understanding of how the human body works.

> **REVISION TIP**
>
> You could be asked about different aspects of medicine, such as prevention or treatment, surgery, and public health. Make sure you know which aspect each development relates to and keep your answers focused on the aspect in question.

Smallpox and inoculation

- Historians believe that smallpox killed more people than any other single infectious disease before the nineteenth century.
- The disease killed 30 per cent of people who caught it, and those who survived would often be left heavily scarred for life.
- **Inoculation** was used to try to protect people from smallpox.

| In Asia in the medieval period, people used a basic form of inoculation to prevent smallpox. They scratched pus or scabs from a smallpox victim onto a healthy person's skin. This gave them a mild dose of the disease, which helped them build up resistance against the full disease. | In the 1720s, inoculation was introduced to Britain by Lady Mary Wortley Montagu. She travelled to Turkey with her family, where she learned about smallpox inoculation, and she had her young son inoculated there. Once back in England, she promoted the technique. | Inoculation slowly became more common in the 1740s and 1750s. However, it had two main problems:
• When someone was inoculated with a mild dose of smallpox, they still became infectious and could spread the disease to others.
• It could be dangerous. If the person being inoculated was accidentally given too large a dose of smallpox, they could suffer badly or even die. |

Edward Jenner and vaccination

Edward Jenner was an English doctor who studied in London with John Hunter. He spent most of his career working as a country doctor in Gloucestershire.

| By chance, Jenner heard stories that milkmaids who caught cowpox were then protected against smallpox. (Cowpox was a much milder version of smallpox that commonly affected cows.) | In 1796, Jenner decided to test this idea by taking pus from a milkmaid's cowpox scar and infecting an 8-year-old boy with it. The boy became mildly ill with cowpox. |
| Jenner repeated this experiment several times before publishing his findings in 1798. None of his patients reacted to the smallpox inoculation after being infected with cowpox. | Six weeks later, Jenner gave the boy the smallpox inoculation. The boy didn't become ill, showing that the dose of cowpox had protected the boy against smallpox. |

Opposition to change

Jenner named his new technique **vaccination** (the Latin word for 'cow' is *vacca*). There was opposition to it because:

- Jenner couldn't explain how his vaccine worked, which made it difficult for others to accept it.
- Many doctors profited from giving smallpox inoculations and didn't want this source of income to end.
- Two doctors in the London Smallpox Hospital carried out tests using cowpox, but their equipment was contaminated and one of their patients died. They believed this showed vaccination wasn't safer than inoculation.
- Some people still argued that as illness came from God, trying to prevent it went against God's will.

However, people eventually realised vaccination was more effective and less dangerous than inoculation.

- By the 1800s, doctors in the USA and Europe were using Jenner's technique.
- In 1853, the British government made smallpox vaccination compulsory.
- By 1980, smallpox was completely eradicated around the world.

Retrieval

Learn the answers to the questions below, then cover the answers column with a piece of paper and write down as many as you can. Check and repeat.

Questions | Answers

#	Question	Answer
1	What effective treatment did Thomas Sydenham introduce to treat anaemia?	Iron
2	Give two reasons why the medicines sold by quacks were popular in the seventeenth and eighteenth centuries.	Two from: they were cheap / they were expertly marketed / they often contained enough alcohol or opium to mask a person's symptoms
3	How many people did the Great Plague kill in London in 1665?	Around 100,000
4	In 1665, what were 'searchers' paid to do?	Identify people suffering from the plague
5	Give two sources of funding for hospitals in the eighteenth century.	Two from: the monarch / businesses / charities / wealthy individuals / private subscription
6	How did most surgeons train in the seventeenth century?	By learning from another surgeon through an apprenticeship
7	Describe the experiment that John Hunter carried out to prove that mercury was an ineffective treatment for gonorrhoea.	He gave some patients mercury pills and others bread pills. He found that all the patients got better, regardless of which pills they took
8	Who introduced inoculation to Britain in the 1720s?	Lady Mary Wortley Montagu
9	In 1796, Edward Jenner infected a boy with cowpox. How did the boy react when he was given the smallpox inoculation?	He didn't become ill
10	Give two reasons why there was opposition to Edward Jenner's new technique of vaccination.	Two from: Jenner couldn't explain how his vaccine worked / many doctors profited from giving smallpox inoculations / two doctors carried out tests using cowpox, but their equipment was contaminated and one of their patients died / some people still argued that trying to prevent illness went against God's will

Previous questions

Use the questions below to check your knowledge from previous chapters.

Questions | Answers

#	Question	Answer
1	What were Lazar houses?	Specialist hospitals for people with leprosy
2	What were gong farmers meant to do with the waste from cesspits?	Take it outside the town walls
3	According to Galen, which organ in the human body made new blood?	The liver

4 Dealing with, and preventing, disease

Practice

Exam-style questions

Study **Source A**.

Source A: A cartoon called 'Time [is] the best doctor' from 1803, by the Scottish cartoonist Isaac Cruikshank. In the cartoon, four doctors are discussing what is wrong with a pregnant woman: one thinks her large stomach is a 'collection of water', another that it's 'wind', a third that it something between the two, and the fourth that it's something that will heal with time. Two doctors wear old-fashioned physician wigs, while two carry surgical instruments.

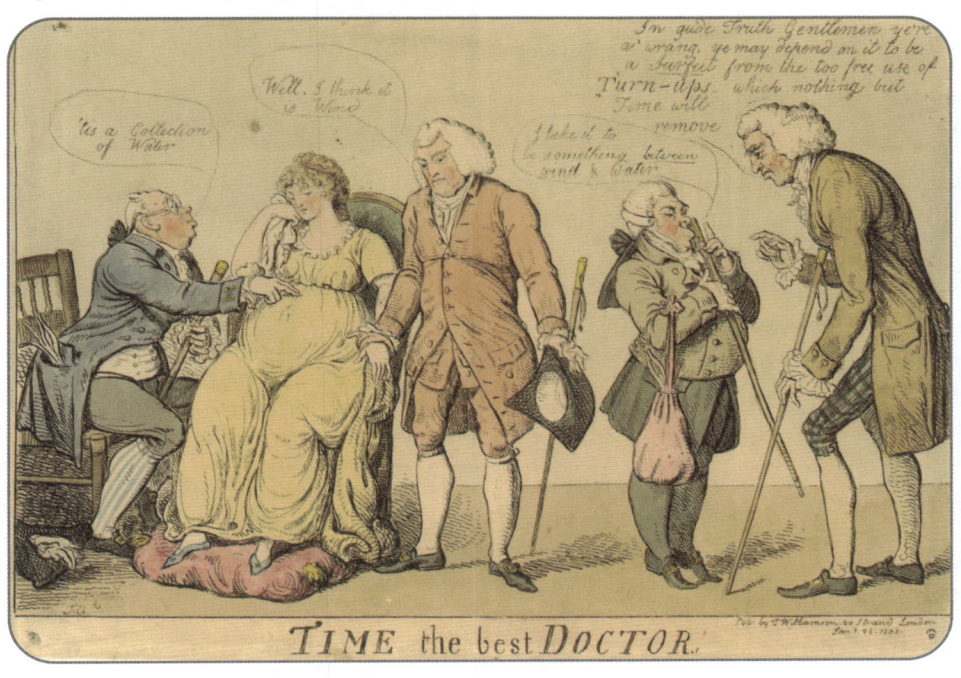

1. How useful is **Source A** to an historian studying eighteenth-century medicine? Explain your answer using **Source A** and your contextual knowledge. (8)

2. Explain the significance of hospitals in the development of medicine. (8)

3. Explain **two ways** in which medieval treatments and treatments in the eighteenth century were similar. (8)

4. Has science and technology been the main factor in improving the treatment of disease in Britain? Explain your answer with reference to the role of science and technology and other factors. Use a range of examples from across your study of Health and the people: c1000 to the present day. (16)

EXAM TIP

When we say an event, idea, or person is significant, we mean more than just that it is important. Judging the significance of an event, idea, or person is about looking at the impact at the time and whether there was a long-term impact. We might, for example, say something is more significant if it not only made an impact at the time, but there were long-lasting impacts too. You may wish to revisit this question once you have revised later periods.

Knowledge

PART THREE: A revolution in medicine

5 Advances in medical science

Microbes and spontaneous generation

- Microscopes were first used to identify **microbes** (germs) in the late seventeenth century, but there was no understanding yet that these caused disease.
- Instead, a popular theory in the eighteenth century was **spontaneous generation**: the idea that microbes were created by decaying matter (rotten food or human waste).
- Scientists incorrectly believed that disease caused microbes, rather than the other way around.

Louis Pasteur

In the late 1850s, the French scientist Louis **Pasteur** was asked by a winemaker to help work out why their wine kept going sour. This prompted Pasteur to conduct experiments over several years into why wine and beer often went sour.

> Pasteur used a microscope to show that there were bacteria (a type of microbe) in spoiled wine. He believed this was causing the wine to turn sour.

> Pasteur proved that heating the wine killed the bacteria. This heating process could therefore be used to prevent wine from souring. (This process is known as '**pasteurisation**' and is still used today for milk.)

> Pasteur disproved the idea of spontaneous generation. He showed that microbes are present in the air, and that some of them can cause decay. This is called **Germ Theory**. Pasteur published his theory in 1861.

> Pasteur next took some broth and boiled it in two swan-necked flasks. This killed the microbes in the broth. He then broke the neck off one of the flasks. The broth in this flask soured, because it was exposed to microbes in the air. But the broth in the other flask didn't spoil, because the swan-neck prevented microbes in the air getting into the flask.

Robert Koch

Robert **Koch** was a German surgeon, born in 1843.

- Koch took Pasteur's Germ Theory (which proved that microbes in the air caused substances such as beer and wine to turn sour) and linked this to illness in humans.
- In 1876, Koch found a way of staining and growing the specific germ that he thought was responsible for anthrax (a disease that causes sores on the lungs). He then proved the germ caused the disease by injecting it into mice and making them ill. This was the first time the specific germ for a disease had been identified.
- Koch went on to identify the germs that caused **cholera** and tuberculosis (TB). He made important contributions to **microbiology** that helped other scientists identify the germs responsible for other diseases.

Koch's contributions

- Proved that not all microbes are the same: specific germs cause specific diseases.
- Discovered how to use dyes to stain specific microbes, so it was easier to see them under a microscope.
- Developed a technique for growing microbes, to make it easier to study them.
- Developed ways of photographing microbes, so other scientists could study them in detail.

Pasteur and vaccination

The first successful vaccine was created by Jenner in 1796, but Jenner didn't fully understand how it worked. Medical knowledge at the time wasn't advanced enough.

| The work of Pasteur and Koch meant that by the 1880s, it was possible to identify the germs that caused specific diseases. This was important for creating vaccines to protect against those diseases. | In 1879, Pasteur was investigating chicken cholera. By accident, he left some cholera germs out of the refrigerator and his assistant, Charles Chamberland, later injected these old, weakened germs into some chickens. The chickens didn't become ill, even when they were then injected with fresh strong germs. | Pasteur showed that the weakened microbes built up the chickens' **immunity** against cholera. He used this principle to develop vaccines for other diseases, such as anthrax (in 1881) and rabies (1885). |

The impact of Pasteur and Koch's work in Britain

Pasteur and Koch were helped by several factors. They were well funded by their respective governments, partly because war between Germany and France in 1870–71 meant both nations were interested in medical research that could help save soldiers' lives. Pasteur and Koch were also hard-working and strong-willed. All these factors helped their research and led to important advances.

However, many scientists and doctors in Britain were sceptical of Pasteur's Germ Theory and Koch's work.

- They found it hard to believe that microscopic germs could harm something as large and advanced as a human. For example, the surgeon Henry Bastian was a prominent critic who wrote many articles defending spontaneous generation.
- Pasteur did have some supporters in Britain. One was scientist John Tyndall, who carried out experiments to show that microbes exist in the air. Another was surgeon William Cheyne, who translated Koch's work into English. A third was the doctor William Roberts, who used Koch's work to draw attention to the role of germs in human infections.

- Due to accumulating scientific evidence, and people such as Tyndall and Cheyne communicating and defending it, Germ Theory became widely accepted in Britain in the 1880s. How did this affect ordinary people?

Pasteur and Koch's work led to the creation of vaccines and chemical cures, making the prevention and treatment of disease much more effective. For example, a vaccine for TB was developed in the 1910s and for polio in the 1950s.

Germ Theory led to the development of **antiseptic** and then **aseptic** surgery, which greatly reduced infections and made surgery safer.

It took time for Germ Theory to be accepted and to influence medical practice. Meanwhile, some doctors in the nineteenth century still believed to some extent in the theory of the four humours. Treatments still included natural remedies, bloodletting, purging, and rest.

Paul Ehrlich and magic bullets

Paul **Ehrlich** was a German scientist who worked with Koch on using dyes to stain specific bacteria to make them easier to identify.

| Instead of using chemicals to stain bacteria, Ehrlich thought that he could use them to kill bacteria. A chemical that can seek out and kill specific germs inside a person without harming them in any other way is called a '**magic bullet**'. | Ehrlich focused his research on syphilis. In 1909, Ehrlich's assistant Sahachiro Hata found that the 606th chemical compound Ehrlich had tried was a success. It was named Salvarsan 606, and was the first chemical cure for any disease. | Ehrlich's research inspired other scientists to search for magic bullets. In 1932, the German scientist Gerhard Domagk found the second magic bullet: a chemical called Prontosil that killed the bacterium *streptococcal*, which caused blood poisoning. |

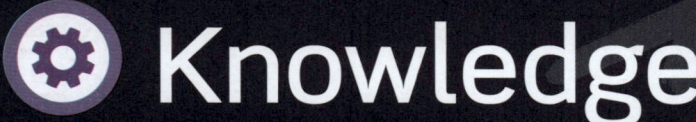

Knowledge — PART THREE: A revolution in medicine

5 Advances in medical science

Anaesthetics in surgery

- Before the nineteenth century, surgeons had no safe, effective anaesthetic: it was hard to control or stop pain during surgery, and patients had to be conscious.
- This meant surgery had to be hurried and it was often imprecise. It was also impossible to carry out complicated internal surgery.
- Natural substances such as mandrake and opium had been used since the Middle Ages to dull pain, but it was hard to distinguish an effective dose from a lethal one.

Three important anaesthetic substances were discovered during the nineteenth century.

Nitrous oxide

- In 1795, the British doctor Thomas Beddoes and his assistant Humphrey Davy experimented with inhaling nitrous oxide ('laughing gas'), but didn't recognise its medical value.
- In 1844, the American dentist Horace Wells tried using nitrous oxide as an anaesthetic when extracting teeth. Following this, it became used in surgery.
- It is still sometimes used in surgery and dentistry today, but it can cause serious side effects and is environmentally damaging.

Ether

- In 1842, the American dentist William Clark tried using ether as an anaesthetic. Others experimented with it too, and it became popular in Britain after Robert Liston gave it to a patient in 1846 when he amputated one of their legs.
- Ether was effective, but had drawbacks: it was difficult to inhale, caused vomiting, and was highly flammable.
- Ether is still sometimes used in less economically developed countries due to its low cost, but it has been replaced in more economically developed countries by more effective anaesthetics.

Chloroform

- In 1847, the Scottish doctor James **Simpson** and his friends tried experimenting with different substances, and found that inhaling chloroform made them unconscious.
- Many doctors were initially wary of using chloroform because too big a dose could kill a patient. For example, a teenage girl died in 1848 during an operation to remove her toenail.
- In 1853, the English doctor John Snow administered chloroform to Queen Victoria during the birth to her eighth child. The Queen wrote that 'the effect was soothing, quieting, and delightful beyond measure', and chloroform became a popular anaesthetic.
- Chloroform is no longer used today as it can cause serious side effects, including heart failure.

REVISION TIP

Being able to use key terms correctly in your exam will improve your answers. Check that you understand the scientific and medical terms in this book and can spell them accurately. You can test your understanding of key terms by writing definitions for them and comparing your answers to the online glossary.

Antiseptics in surgery

- Historians believe that the introduction of anaesthetics to British surgery initially increased the number of patients dying.
- This was because operations no longer had to be as quick as possible to spare patients pain. Instead, surgeons could perform more complicated and invasive procedures, which led to more infections.
- Wounds could easily become infected and infections were often fatal. Surgeons didn't yet know that germs caused infections, so they saw no need to keep operating theatres clean.
- Joseph **Lister**, a Professor of Surgery in Glasgow, helped solve this problem by starting to use antiseptics in surgery.

> Lister realised that his operations went well as long as the wound was kept free from infection.

> He read about Pasteur's Germ Theory and wondered if he could use a chemical to kill any bacteria that might infect a wound during surgery.

> In 1865, he started using carbolic acid as an antiseptic, soaking bandages in the chemical before applying them to a wound. He also sprayed carbolic acid on his hands and on the equipment used during an operation.

> The mortality rate in Lister's own surgery fell from 46 per cent to 15 per cent.

> Lister published his results in 1867, and gave lectures to doctors on his findings.

There was some opposition to Lister's approach because:

- it relied on accepting Pasteur's Germ Theory, but many doctors still believed in spontaneous generation
- it slowed surgery down, and speed was still important in preventing blood loss
- carbolic acid was unpleasant to use: it irritated surgeons' hands, eyes, and lungs
- Lister was very critical of other surgeons, which made them defensive of their own approaches.

However, other surgeons started to copy his ideas and this contributed to making surgery safer.

Aseptic surgery

Surgeons built on Lister's ideas to develop aseptic surgery in the 1890s. Instead of using antiseptics (such as carbolic acid) to kill germs in the operating theatre, aseptic surgery aimed to create a sterile environment where germs are excluded from the start.

One development that contributed to this was the introduction of surgical gloves.

- William Halsted was an American surgeon who used antiseptics in his operating theatre. In 1889, he asked a tyre company to make thin rubber gloves for nurse Caroline Hampton, as the skin on her hands reacted badly to the antiseptics.
- Although the gloves weren't initially introduced to improve cleanliness, Halstad and other surgeons soon found that they helped to reduce infections.

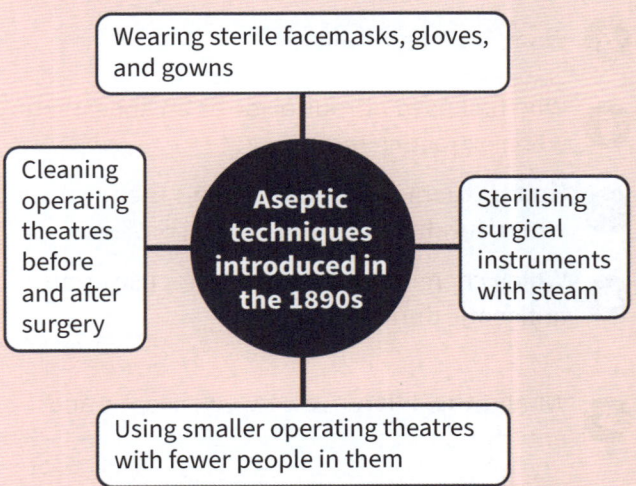

Aseptic techniques introduced in the 1890s:
- Wearing sterile facemasks, gloves, and gowns
- Cleaning operating theatres before and after surgery
- Sterilising surgical instruments with steam
- Using smaller operating theatres with fewer people in them

Key terms — Make sure you can write a definition for these key terms

microbe   spontaneous generation
Pasteur   pasteurisation   Germ Theory
Koch   cholera   microbiology
immunity   antiseptic   aseptic
Ehrlich   magic bullet
Simpson   Lister

5 Knowledge

Retrieval

Learn the answers to the questions below, then cover the answers column with a piece of paper and write down as many as you can. Check and repeat.

Questions / Answers

1. **What is the theory of spontaneous generation?**
   Microbes are created by decaying matter, such as rotten food or human waste

2. **Describe how Pasteur used two swan-necked flasks to show that microbes are present in the air.**
   Pasteur took some broth and boiled it in two swan-necked flasks. This killed the microbes in the broth. He then broke the neck off one of the flasks. The broth in this flask soured, because it was exposed to microbes in the air. But the broth in the other flask didn't spoil, because the swan-neck prevented microbes in the air getting into the flask

3. **In 1876, how did Koch prove that he had found the germ that causes anthrax?**
   By injecting it into mice and making them ill

4. **When Charles Chamberland injected chickens with old, weakened cholera germs, how did the chickens react?**
   The chickens didn't become ill, even when they were then injected with fresh strong germs

5. **What is a magic bullet?**
   A chemical that can seek out and kill specific germs inside a person without harming them in any other way

6. **Who first used nitrous oxide as an anaesthetic when extracting teeth?**
   American dentist Horace Wells

7. **How did James Simpson and his friends react when they first tried inhaling chloroform?**
   It made them unconscious

8. **Which chemical did Jospeh Lister use as an antiseptic during surgery?**
   Carbolic acid

9. **What is the difference between aseptic and antiseptic surgery?**
   Antiseptic surgery uses antiseptics to kill germs in the operating theatre. Aseptic surgery aims to create a sterile environment where germs are excluded from the start

Previous questions

Use the questions below to check your knowledge from previous chapters.

Questions / Answers

1. **One way the Black Death spread was through infected people coughing and sneezing. What was the other way?**
   Fleas that were infected with *Yersinia pestis* biting people

2. **What was the title of Vesalius' famous book, published in 1543?**
   On the Fabric of the Human Body

3. **In 1796, Edward Jenner infected a boy with cowpox. How did the boy react when he was given the smallpox inoculation?**
   He didn't become ill

5 Advances in medical science

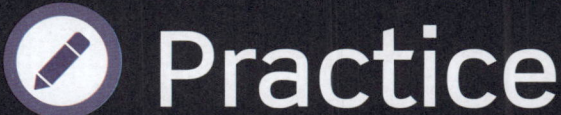

Practice

5

Exam-style questions

Study **Source A**.

Source A: An engraving published in the book *Antiseptic Surgery: Its Principles, Practice, History and Results* by William Cheyne in 1882. The engraving shows surgeons performing an operation using carbolic spray as an antiseptic. Cheyne was Joseph Lister's deputy surgeon.

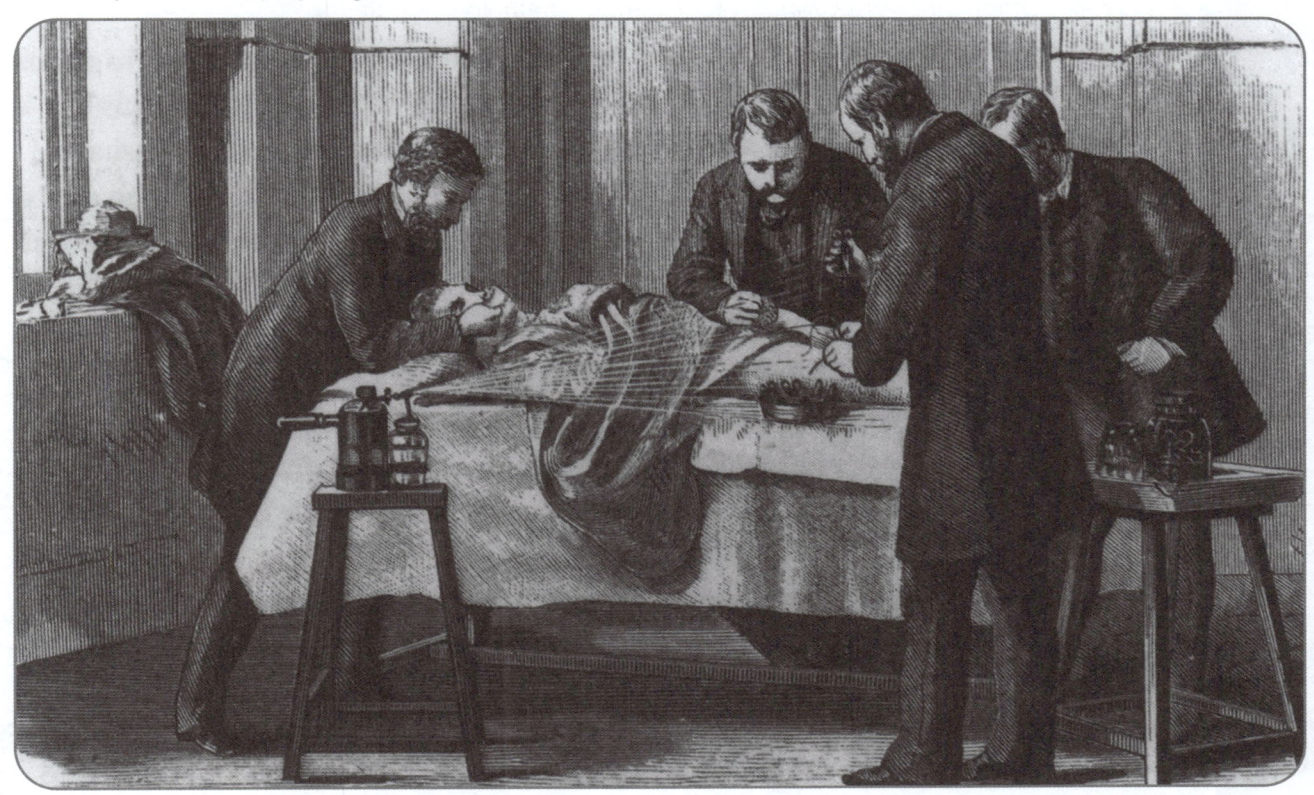

1. How useful is **Source A** to an historian studying surgery in the nineteenth century? Explain your answer using **Source A** and your contextual knowledge. **(8)**

2. Explain the significance of Germ Theory. **(8)**

3. Explain **two ways** in which the discovery of new medical ideas in the Renaissance and in the nineteenth century were similar. **(8)**

4. Has chance been the main factor in the development of medicine? Explain your answer with reference to the role of chance and other factors. Use a range of examples from across your study of Health and the people: c1000 to the present day. **(16)**

EXAM TIP

Question 4 requires you to draw on a range of examples from across the periods of your study. A strong answer will give examples from at least three different periods, so try to include examples from all the periods covered so far. Examples of chance influencing the development of medicine (remember you need to write about other factors too) could include Paré, Jenner, Pasteur, and Simpson. You can revisit this question when you have revised the modern period as well.

Knowledge — PART THREE: A revolution in medicine

6 Improvements in public health

Public health problems in industrial Britain

The Industrial Revolution led to large advances in technology and transport between 1750 and 1900. Goods were made in factories with the help of machines, rather than by hand at home.

- People left the countryside to take jobs in the new factories that were being built in urban areas across Britain. Cities grew rapidly, for example Sheffield's population increased more than ten-fold between 1750 and 1860.
- Cheap back-to-back housing was quickly built to accommodate these new workers.
- Overcrowding and poor sanitation meant that diseases such as typhoid and TB spread quickly. The average age of death was around 40, as many people's health declined.

Reasons for poor public health in towns and cities in industrial Britain:

- Few houses had toilets. Some families simply used a bucket that they emptied into the street.
- Many houses were overcrowded, with whole families living in a single room.
- There were some public toilets (deep holes with wooden sheds over them), but these were shared between houses.
- People didn't yet know what caused disease or how to avoid falling ill.
- There were some water pumps in the streets, but these usually took polluted water from the local river or pond.
- There were no rubbish collections, street cleaners, or sewers.
- Sewage in the streets was washed into nearby rivers, which is where most families washed their clothes and bathed.

Cholera epidemics

In 1831, cholera arrived in Britain and killed around 50,000 people.

- There was no cure and no one understood what caused it: many people believed it was spread by miasma.
- There were further outbreaks in the following decades, and the 1837–38 outbreak pushed the government into action.
- During the 1854 outbreak, the English doctor John Snow discovered that cholera was spread through dirty water.

John Snow worked on Broad Street, in Soho, London.

- In 1854, over 700 people living in or near Broad Street died of cholera within ten days.
- Snow investigated the deaths and found that all the victims had got their water from the Broad Street water pump.
- Snow persuaded the local council to remove the handle of the water pump so people could no longer use it.
- Snow proved that cholera wasn't carried through the air and spread by miasma. Instead he showed that it is often spread through contaminated water.
- Snow investigated further and found that a street toilet next to the pump had a cracked lining. Human waste from cholera sufferers was trickling into the drinking water.
- There were no more deaths from cholera in the area.

Government involvement and public health reformers

In the early nineteenth century, the government took a *laissez-faire* approach to public health. Many believed the government shouldn't interfere in people's lives and force them to change.

During the course of the nineteenth century, the government was prompted to become more involved in improving public health. This was mainly due to:

- the ongoing cholera epidemics
- a growing awareness that poor living conditions led to poor health
- working-class men being given the vote in 1867. (Politicians realised that improving living conditions for the working classes would gain them votes.)

Report on the Sanitary Conditions of the Labouring Population of Great Britain

Prompted by the cholera outbreaks in the 1830s, the government set up an inquiry in 1839 to investigate health and living conditions among the working classes in Britain.

- It was led by Edwin Chadwick, a public health reformer. After two years of research, Chadwick published his report in 1842. Thousands of free copies were given out.
- Chadwick highlighted the link between poor living conditions and poor life expectancy. His recommendations included cleaning rubbish from the streets, providing a clean water supply, and installing new sewers.

1842

The Great Stink and Bazalgette's sewers

In London in the early 1800s, a lot of sewage and waste ended up in the Thames (the main river).

- In the summer of 1858, a heatwave meant the water level of the Thames dropped, exposing a lot of the sewage and waste. The smell was so bad that the Houses of Parliament next to the river were closed.
- The Great Stink prompted the government to ask the engineer Joseph Bazalgette to build a network of technologically advanced underground sewers across London. Bazalgette was given £3 million (worth around £300 million today) to build the sewers.
- The sewers were finished in 1866 and, after this, cholera never returned to London.

1848

First Public Health Act

Many politicians were dismissive of Chadwick's ideas and believed they would be too expensive to implement. However, further cholera outbreaks encouraged the government to act.

- The first Public Health Act (1848) gave local councils the power to clean up their streets and improve facilities – *if* they wanted to, and *if* they paid for it themselves. (Many cities and towns chose not to, but some places like Liverpool and Birmingham did make improvements.)
- The Act established a Central Board of Health to oversee improvements in public health, though this was shut down in 1854 due to resentment at government interference.

1858

1875

Second Public Health Act

After Chadwick's report, Snow's work on cholera, and Pasteur's publication of Germ Theory, it became clear to the government that cleaner towns and cities would improve public health.

- The second Public Health Act (1875) ordered local councils to keep sewers in good condition, supply fresh water, collect rubbish, and appoint a medical officer for each district.
- Partly due to the government's reforms, the average age of death in Britain rose from around 40 to 46 over the course of the nineteenth century.

Key term — Make sure you can write a definition for this key term: *laissez-faire*

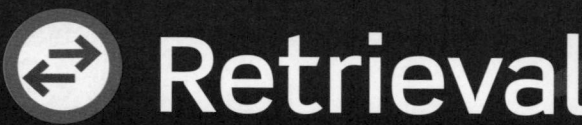

Retrieval

Learn the answers to the questions below, then cover the answers column with a piece of paper and write down as many as you can. Check and repeat.

Questions | Answers

1. Why did the Industrial Revolution lead to overcrowding in towns and cities? — Because people left the countryside to take jobs in the new factories that were being built in urban areas across Britain

2. In the early nineteenth century, where did water pumps in the streets usually take their water from? — From the local river or pond

3. When cholera first arrived in Britain, how did many people think it was spread? — By miasma

4. What was the source of the cholera deaths that John Snow investigated in 1854? — The Broad Street water pump

5. What did John Snow persuade the local council to do once he found the source of the cholera deaths? — Remove the handle of the water pump so people could no longer use it

6. Why did the government take a *laissez-faire* approach to public health in the early nineteenth century? — Many believed the government shouldn't interfere in people's lives and force them to change

7. Who wrote *Report on the Sanitary Conditions of the Labouring Population of Great Britain*? — Edwin Chadwick

8. What caused the Great Stink in 1858? — A heatwave meant the water level of the Thames dropped, exposing a lot of the sewage and waste in the river

9. What did the Great Stink prompt the government to do? — To ask the engineer Joseph Bazalgette to build a network of technologically advanced underground sewers across London

10. Give two things the Second Public Health Act ordered local councils to do. — Two from: keep sewers in good condition / supply fresh water / collect rubbish / appoint a medical officer for each district

Previous questions

Use the questions below to check your knowledge from previous chapters.

Questions | Answers

1. In which year did the Black Death reach England? — 1348

2. Who introduced inoculation to Britain in the 1720s? — Lady Mary Wortley Montagu

3. What is the theory of spontaneous generation? — Microbes are created by decaying matter, such as rotten food or human waste

6 Improvements in public health

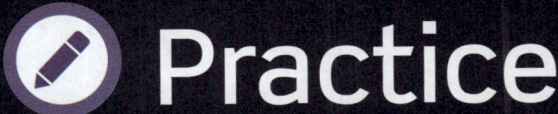

Practice

6

Exam-style questions

Study **Source A**.

Source A: An 1858 cartoon from the British satirical magazine *Punch*, published in July at the time of the Great Stink. The cartoon is called 'Father Thames introduces his children, Diphtheria, Scrofula and Cholera, to London.' Diphtheria, scrofula, and cholera are all serious contagious diseases.

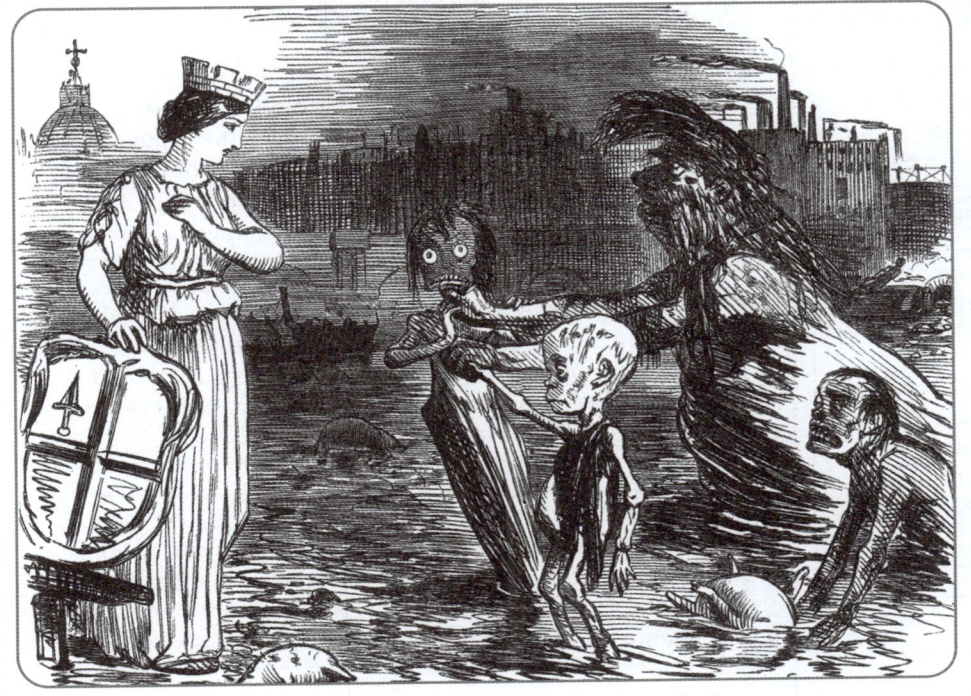

> **SOURCE TIP**
>
> A satirical magazine features humorous cartoons and stories that aim to make people laugh, often by poking fun at people in power. Consider this aim when thinking about how useful the cartoon is as a source of historical information. Remember a source can be *unreliable* and still be *useful*.

1. How useful is **Source A** to an historian studying public health in the nineteenth century? Explain your answer using **Source A** and your contextual knowledge. **(8)**

2. Explain the significance of the British government's public health reforms in the nineteenth century. **(8)**

> **EXAM TIP**
>
> Remember, for a full answer to this question, you will also need to refer to public health in the modern period. This will allow you to consider the *long-term* significance of the reforms, as well as their short-term impact. Come back to the question when you have revised the modern period.

3. Explain **two ways** in which public health in the Middle Ages and public health in the nineteenth century were similar. **(8)**

4. Has science and technology been the main factor in improving public health in Britain? Explain your answer with reference to the role of science and technology and other factors. Use a range of examples from across your study of Health and the people: c1000 to the present day. **(16)**

Knowledge — PART FOUR: Modern medicine

7 Modern treatment of disease

Penicillin

Before **penicillin** became widely available in the 1940s, even minor infections could still be deadly.

Alexander Fleming discovers penicillin

- Alexander **Fleming** was a Scottish scientist who studied the treatment of wounded soldiers during the First World War. He was determined to find a better way to treat infected wounds.
- In 1928, Fleming went on holiday and left *staphylococcus* bacteria in a **Petri dish** sitting next to an open window in his lab.
- When Fleming returned, he found that mould had grown in the Petri dish by chance. The *staphylococcus* bacteria next to the mould had been killed.
- Fleming found that the 'juice' from the mould had killed the bacteria and he named it penicillin.
- Fleming published his findings in 1929, but his work received little attention.

Howard Florey and Ernest Chain develop penicillin

- In the 1930s, the scientists Florey and Chain were researching natural substances that could kill germs. Inspired by Fleming's article on penicillin, they applied to the British government for funding to research it, but received only £25 (worth around £1,300 today). Despite this, they found a way to grow and purify a small amount of penicillin.
- After successfully testing the penicillin on mice, in 1941 they gave it to policeman Albert Alexander. A small cut on his cheek had become infected and he was very ill. Alexander started to recover, but after five days the penicillin ran out and he died a few weeks later.
- Florey realised that penicillin needed to be mass-produced. In July 1941, he travelled to the USA to meet with the US government, which was keen to mass-produce penicillin because so many US soldiers were dying from infected wounds during the Second World War.
- The US government paid several large pharmaceutical companies to mass-produce penicillin. By the end of the war in 1945, enough penicillin was being produced to treat millions of people.

Historians estimate that 12 to 15 per cent of wounded British and American soldiers would have died during the Second World War without being given penicillin.

Penicillin is still commonly used to treat bacterial infections and is estimated to have saved hundreds of millions of lives.

The growth of the pharmaceutical industry

The pharmaceutical industry develops and produces drugs for use in medicine and health care.

- In the early nineteenth century, drugs were mostly produced by small businesses.
- Businesses were able to scale up towards the end of the century due to advances in science and technology, such as the invention of a tablet-making machine in 1843 and a gelatine pill capsule in 1875.
- The pharmaceutical industry grew substantially during the Second World War because of the huge demand for penicillin. Government funding was an important source of finance at this time.
- Today the industry is one of the biggest in the world.

New treatments and new diseases

Many important medical advances have been made since the start of the twentieth century. The timeline below gives some of the most important ones.

- **1950** — Canadian surgeon William Bigelow performs the first open-heart surgery to repair a hole in a baby's heart.
- **1953** — Francis Crick and James Watson map out the structure of **DNA**, building on Rosalind Franklin's work to **X-ray** DNA. This leads to developments such as gene therapy and genetic screening.
- **1973** — British scientist Geoff Hounsfield invents the CAT scanner, which uses X-ray images from many angles to build up a 3D image of the inside of the body.
- **1977** — Raymond Damadian carries out the first full-body scan of a patient using an MRI scanner. This produces detailed images of the inside of the body.
- **1978** — Louise Brown is the first baby to be born using IVF. IVF helps people with fertility problems to have a baby, by fertilising an egg with a sperm outside the human body.
- **2003** — The human genome (all the genes that make up human DNA) is fully mapped out. This research helps develop understanding of genetic diseases and how to treat them.

While improvements in medicine have helped to greatly reduce the impact of some diseases (particularly infectious diseases like TB), other diseases have become more common over the past century, such as heart disease, cancer, and Alzheimer's.

These 'new' diseases have become more common partly because of a general increase in poor diet, obesity, and habits such as smoking and drinking. The fact people are living longer also means more people are suffering from age-related diseases like Alzheimer's.

Antibiotic resistance

Over recent decades, some bacteria have evolved to become resistant to **antibiotics** (such as penicillin). These antibiotic-resistant bacteria are sometimes called **superbugs**. One example is MRSA, first reported in a British study in 1961.

One reason why superbugs are emerging is because antibiotics have been overused. For example, they have been used for illnesses like colds or flu (which are caused by viruses, not bacteria, so are not affected by antibiotics).

This has led to some governments and health services trying to use antibiotics in a more restrained way. It has also prompted pharmaceutical companies to look for new antibiotics that can kill superbugs.

Alternative treatments

Some people use alternative treatments, such as **aromatherapy**, **acupuncture**, **homeopathy**, and **hypnotherapy**. They use these in addition to, or instead of, the mainstream medicine offered by their healthcare system. These alternative therapies typically have less rigorous scientific evidence to back them up than conventional medicine.

However, some alternative therapies do have scientific studies supporting their effectiveness, and some (such as acupuncture) are available through the **NHS**.

Key terms — Make sure you can write a definition for these key terms:

penicillin, Fleming, Petri dish, DNA, X-ray, antibiotic, superbug, aromatherapy, acupuncture, homeopathy, hypnotherapy, NHS

Retrieval

Learn the answers to the questions below, then cover the answers column with a piece of paper and write down as many as you can. Check and repeat.

Questions | Answers

1. When Alexander Fleming discovered penicillin, which bacteria was he investigating? — *Staphylococcus*

2. Which two scientists found a way to grow and purify penicillin? — Howard Florey and Ernest Chain

3. What happened to Albert Alexander when he was given penicillin in 1941? — Alexander started to recover, but after five days the penicillin ran out and he died a few weeks later

4. Why was the US government keen to mass-produce penicillin in the early 1940s? — Because so many US soldiers were dying from infected wounds during the Second World War

5. Why were pharmaceutical businesses able to scale up at the end of the nineteenth century? — Because of advances in science and technology, such as the invention of a tablet-making machine in 1843 and a gelatine pill capsule in 1875

6. Which three scientists contributed to the understanding of the DNA model? — Rosalind Franklin, Francis Crick, and James Watson

7. What does a CAT scanner do? — Uses X-ray images from many angles to build up a 3D image of the inside of the body

8. By when was the human genome fully mapped out? — 2003

9. What are superbugs? — Bacteria that have evolved to become resistant to the antibiotics that are used to kill them

10. Why is it ineffective to use antibiotics for colds or flu? — Because these illnesses are caused by viruses, not bacteria, so are not affected by antibiotics

11. Name three types of alternative treatments. — Three from: aromatherapy / acupuncture / homeopathy / hypnotherapy

Previous questions

Use the questions below to check your knowledge from previous chapters.

Questions | Answers

1. How did most surgeons train in the seventeenth century? — By learning from another surgeon through an apprenticeship

2. In 1876, how did Koch prove that he had found the germ that causes anthrax? — By injecting it into mice and making them ill

3. When cholera first arrived in Britain, how did many people think it was spread? — By miasma

7 Modern treatment of disease

Practice

Exam-style questions

Study **Source A**.

Source A: A 2007 cartoon by Steve Greenberg, an American cartoonist. The cartoon was first published in a daily newspaper in California.

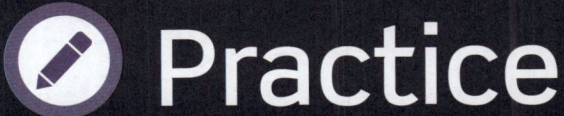

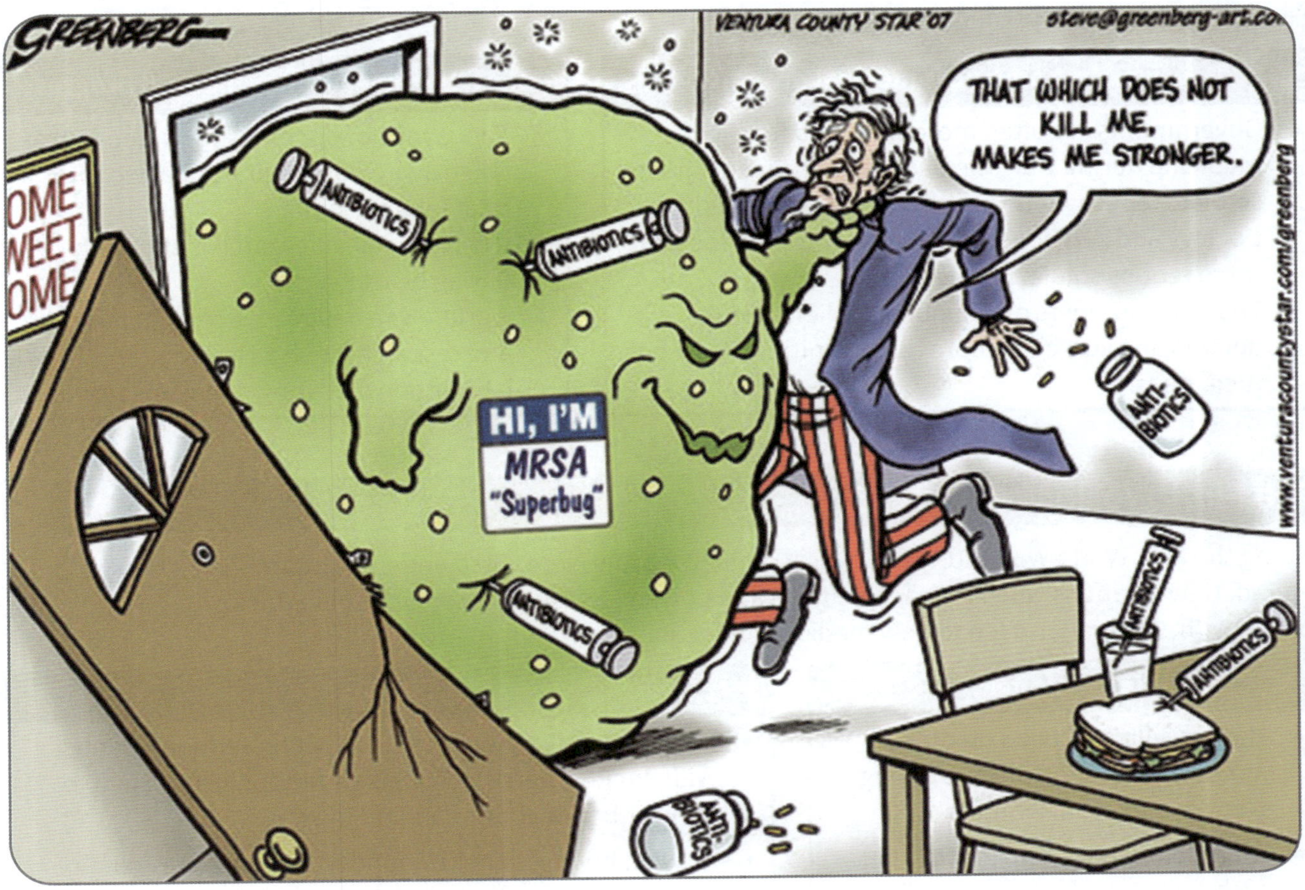

1. How useful is **Source A** to an historian studying modern medicine? Explain your answer using **Source A** and your contextual knowledge. **(8)**

2. Explain the significance of the work of Howard Florey and Ernest Chain. **(8)**

3. Explain **two ways** in which the treatment of illness and disease in the seventeenth century and the treatment of illness and disease in the twenty-first century were similar. **(8)**

4. Has the role of government been the main factor in improving the treatment of disease? Explain your answer with reference to the role of the government and other factors. Use a range of examples from across your study of Health and the people: c1000 to the present day. **(16)**

> **EXAM TIP**
>
> Structure your answer by first writing about the factor mentioned in the question (the government). You could mention how government funding helped the work of scientists like Pasteur, Koch, Florey, and Chain, as well as the NHS (see Chapter 9). Then consider other factors (such as the role of the individual, or technology and science). Finish with a short conclusion where you say which factor you think has been most influential and why.

Knowledge

PART FOUR: Modern medicine

8 The impact of war and technology on surgery

The contribution of war to medicine

Medicine tends to develop at a faster rate in wartime than in peacetime, and the twentieth century was dominated by global war on an unprecedented scale. Wartime can also disrupt medical progress.

How wartime advances medical progress	How wartime hinders medical progress
✓ Governments are often more willing to fund medicine during wartime because they need injured soldiers to recover and return to the battlefield. ✓ Doctors and surgeons work hard to develop ideas to try to reduce soldiers' suffering. ✓ The huge numbers of wounded soldiers give doctors and surgeons more opportunities to test out their ideas.	✗ Thousands of doctors and surgeons are taken away from their normal work to treat injured soldiers. ✗ A lot of medical research is stopped during wartime. ✗ Warfare can destroy places of learning and research (such as libraries and laboratories), halting or erasing research.

The First World War

During the First World War (1914–18), over 10 million people were killed and many more injured. New weapons, such as machine guns and poison gas, meant new types of injuries to deal with. The war also led to new medical innovations.

Plastic surgery
- Harold Gillies focused on **plastic surgery** to treat soldiers suffering from severe facial wounds.
- Gillies pioneered **skin graft** techniques, and is recognised as being one of the first surgeons to consider a patient's appearance when treating wounds.

X-rays
- X-rays were discovered in 1895 by the German scientist Wilhelm Roentgen. Hospitals were soon using them to look for broken bones and bullets.
- In 1914, hoping to help wounded soldiers, the French scientist Marie Curie invented a portable X-ray machine.
- This meant X-ray images could be taken near the battlefield. The images helped surgeons locate bullets or **shrapnel** in a soldier's body before operating on them.

Blood transfusions
- In 1901, Austrian scientist Karl Landsteiner discovered three of the four blood groups, and doctors realised that blood transfusions only worked if the blood groups involved matched.
- However, blood clotted quickly outside the body. A donor's blood had to be taken and given immediately to the receiver.
- In 1914, the Belgian doctor Albert Hustin discovered that glucose and sodium citrate stopped blood from clotting on contact with air. This meant it could be stored for a few days.

Other developments
- By the end of the First World War, 'shell shock' became officially recognised. Known today as PTSD, it is the result of psychological damage from the mental strain of trauma.
- Surgeons cut away dead or infected tissue (excision) and soaked wounds in salty (saline) solutions to help prevent infection.
- The Keller-Blake Splint was developed to help broken leg bones knit together more securely. It is still used today.

The Second World War

At least 35 million people died during the Second World War (1939–45) and millions more were injured. As with the First World War, doctors and scientists worked hard to improve treatments for the wounded.

- Blood banks were improved. These collected and stored blood in the large quantities needed by army surgeons. This led to the British National Blood Transfusion Service opening in 1946.

- Penicillin was mass-produced to help cure infections that could have previously been fatal.

- Advances in plastic surgery continued to be made. Doctor Archibald McIndoe (a cousin of Harold Gillies) improved skin graft techniques while treating soldiers with severe burns and facial wounds.

- Heart surgery continued to improve. Surgeon Dwight Harken became an expert at removing bullets and shrapnel from the heart. Many surgeons came to watch and learn from him.

Modern surgical methods

Surgery has continued to improve so more complicated operations can be carried out safely and effectively. Four key developments are outlined below.

Transplants

- An organ transplant involves replacing a damaged human organ with a healthy one.
- Doctors began experimenting with organ transplants in the eighteenth century.
- The first successful organ transplant took place in 1954. A twin donated one of his kidneys to his brother, who had chronic kidney failure.
- Advances in science and medicine have since helped make transplants safer. For example, the development of **immunosuppressant drugs** in the 1980s helped to prevent a patient's immune system rejecting their new organ.

Laser surgery

- **Laser surgery** uses lasers (a type of powerful light beam) instead of surgical instruments (like scalpels) to carry out surgical procedures. It can be more reliable and precise than surgery carried out by hand.
- Laser surgery was first used in an eye operation in 1987 by the doctor Stephen Trokel.
- It is still commonly used in eye surgery. It is also used to help clear blocked arteries, and to remove tumours and ulcers.

Radiation therapy

- After X-rays were discovered in 1895, **radiation therapy** started to be used to treat cancer and other diseases. It uses high-energy radiation to shrink tumours and kill cancer cells.
- Scientific advances mean radiation can now be delivered more precisely, so it harms less of the body.
- Around half of all cancer patients today receive some type of radiation therapy.

Keyhole surgery

- In 1910, Swedish surgeon Hans Christian Jacobaeus performed one of the first operations using **keyhole surgery**.
- Keyhole surgery enables surgeons to access the inside of the body without making large cuts in the skin. Instead, tiny cameras and instruments are inserted into the body through small cuts in the skin.
- It helps patients recover faster after operations and leaves less scarring.
- The technique is used today for a wide range of surgeries, such as brain surgery, heart surgery, and kidney transplants.

Key terms — Make sure you can write a definition for these key terms: plastic surgery, skin graft, shrapnel, immunosuppressant drug, laser surgery, radiation therapy, keyhole surgery

Retrieval

Learn the answers to the questions below, then cover the answers column with a piece of paper and write down as many as you can. Check and repeat.

Questions | Answers

#	Question	Answer
1	Why are governments often more willing to fund medicine during wartime?	Because they need injured soldiers to recover and return to the battlefield
2	What type of soldiers did Harold Gillies treat?	Soldiers suffering from severe facial wounds
3	Who invented the mobile X-ray machine?	Marie Curie
4	Why was the mobile X-ray machine useful in the First World War?	X-ray images could be taken near the battlefield. The images helped surgeons locate bullets or shrapnel in a soldier's body before operating on them
5	Why was the discovery of blood groups in 1901 important for safe blood transfusions?	Because a blood transfusion only works if the blood groups involved match
6	What stops blood from clotting on contact with air? It was discovered in 1914.	Glucose and sodium nitrate
7	Which drug was mass-produced during the Second World War to cure infections?	Penicillin
8	What was Dwight Harken an expert at removing, and from where?	Bullets and shrapnel from the heart
9	Why does having immunosuppressant drugs help to make transplants safer?	Because they help to prevent a patient's immune system rejecting the new organ
10	When was laser surgery first used in an eye operation?	1987
11	How does radiation therapy work?	It uses high-energy radiation to shrink tumours and kill cancer cells
12	What does keyhole surgery involve?	Tiny cameras and instruments are inserted into the body through small cuts in the skin

Previous questions

Use the questions below to check your knowledge from previous chapters.

Questions | Answers

#	Question	Answer
1	How did Paré treat gunshot wounds when he ran out of hot oil during a battle in 1537?	He just smeared the wounds with a cream of rose oil, egg white, and turpentine
2	Why did the government take a *laissez-faire* approach to public health in the early nineteenth century?	Many believed the government shouldn't interfere in people's lives and force them to change
3	What happened to Albert Alexander when he was given penicillin in 1941?	Alexander started to recover, but after five days the penicillin ran out and he died a few weeks later

8 The impact of war and technology on surgery

Practice

8

Exam-style questions

Study **Source A**.

Source A: A poster used by the American government between 1941 and 1944. The poster was used during the Second World War to encourage people working in pharmaceutical companies.

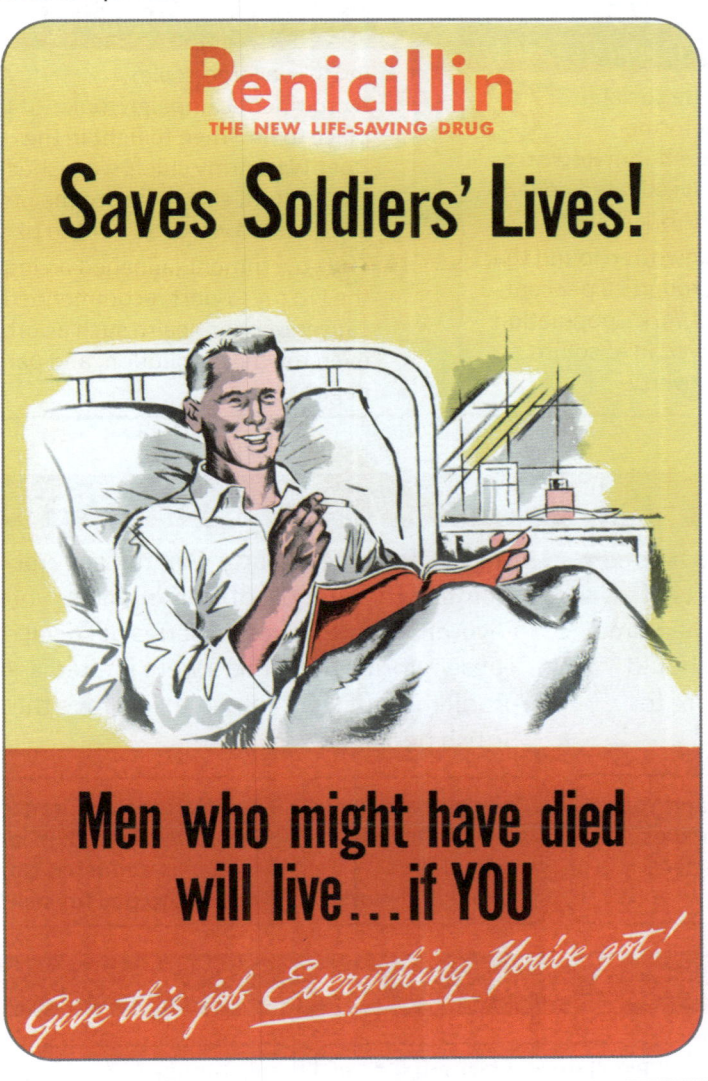

1. How useful is **Source A** to an historian studying modern developments in the treatment of disease? Explain your answer using **Source A** and your contextual knowledge. **(8)**

2. Explain the significance of modern surgical methods in the development of medicine. **(8)**

3. Explain **two ways** in which surgery during the twentieth century and surgery during the nineteenth century were similar. **(8)**

4. Has war been the main factor in improving the treatment of disease in Britain? Explain your answer with reference to the role of war and other factors. Use a range of examples from across your study of Health and the people: c1000 to the present day. **(16)**

> **EXAM TIP**
>
> Remember that you need to write about two similarities between these different periods. Consider surgical techniques or procedures that had similar goals, such as the goal of reducing the risk of dying from infection (whether by using carbolic acid or penicillin).

Knowledge

PART FOUR: Modern medicine

9 Modern public health

Booth, Rowntree, and the Boer War

Between 1899 and 1904, three reports were published that highlighted the problems of poverty and poor health in Britain.

1. Life and Labour of the People in London (1889)
- The social reformer Charles **Booth** researched poverty in London.
- Booth found that around 30 per cent of London's population lived in **absolute poverty**. He showed there was a link between poverty and a high death rate.

2. Poverty: A Study of Town Life (1901)
- The social reformer Seebohm **Rowntree** investigated poverty in York in 1900.
- Rowntree found that around 28 per cent of York's population lived in absolute poverty.

3. The Fitzroy Report (1904)
- In 1899, a large-scale recruitment campaign took place to find men to fight in the **Boer War**. Army chiefs were shocked that around 40 per cent of the men who volunteered were too unfit to be soldiers.
- The government launched an inquiry and the Fitzroy Report recommended tackling causes of poor health such as urban overcrowding, pollution, and parental neglect.

Liberal social reforms

Research by Booth, Rowntree, and others helped to spread awareness of the negative effects of poverty and poor health. This happened at a time when many people felt the government should drop its *laissez-faire* approach and do more to look after the vulnerable.

In 1906, the Liberal Party won the general election. To maintain the support of working-class voters, the new government introduced a series of social reforms. These reforms and others were limited and had their problems, but they helped to improve the welfare of British people.

1906 — The School Meals Act introduces free school meals for children living in poverty.

1907 — The government introduces medical examinations for school students.

1908 — The Children and Young Person's Act makes it illegal to neglect children.

1908 — Pensions are introduced for people over 70 years old.

1909 — Job centres are set up to help unemployed people find work.

1909 — The building of back-to-back housing is banned.

1911 — The National Insurance Act introduces health insurance: money is deducted from workers' salaries to pay for sick leave.

The impact of two world wars

British governments continued to try to improve public health, welfare, and housing during the twentieth century. In particular, the two world wars encouraged governments to make more wide-reaching changes:

- People suffered greatly during the wars. They wanted the government to help create a better future for them.
- The wars showed that the government could act quickly to make positive changes. People wanted the government to use this newfound power to help improve their lives.

After the 1919 Housing Act, local councils started building **council housing** for poorer families. This helped to address the housing shortages after the wars. The 1930 Housing Act also encouraged local councils to replace **slum housing** with better-quality housing.

The Beveridge Report and the Welfare State

William Beveridge was a social reformer and Liberal politician. In 1941, he was asked by the government to review the **social services** it provided.

His report *Social Insurance and Allied Services* (which later became known as the Beveridge Report) was published in 1942.

- The report called for a much more comprehensive **Welfare State**. It said that the government should 'take charge of social security from the cradle to the grave', by dealing with the 'five giants' that could ruin a person's life: disease, idleness, ignorance, want, and squalor (poor living conditions).
- The report also recommended setting up a national health service that would provide free healthcare to all.
- The report was very popular and sold over 100,000 copies in its first month of publication.

The creation and development of the NHS

In 1945, a general election was held to decide who would run the country after the war. The Labour Party promised to follow Beveridge's advice and easily won the election.

- Labour's Minister of Health, Aneurin Bevan, was tasked with founding the NHS to provide free healthcare to everyone. It was introduced in 1948.
- The NHS allowed everyone to get free medical advice and treatment. From 1948 to 2019, life expectancy increased by an average of 13 years: the NHS played a major role in this.
- From the 1940s onwards, the Welfare State expanded in other ways too, providing education, housing, childcare, and financial help.

Developments in the NHS

- Treatments have improved as science and technology advances.
- New hospitals have been built and old ones refurbished to try to keep up with growing demand.
- Nationwide vaccination programmes have been introduced, such as for polio in 1958 and measles in 1968.
- The NHS has run public health campaigns to encourage people to make healthy lifestyle choices, such as the '5 A Day' campaign (to encourage people to eat more fruit and vegetables).

The cost of healthcare in the twenty-first century

The NHS is largely funded through taxes. When the NHS opened in 1948, some people argued (and have argued since) that it costs taxpayers too much money.

- By 1951, it had become clear that taxpayers couldn't pay for everything. Charges were introduced for prescriptions, eye care, and dental care.
- In 2022, the government spent £182 billion on the NHS. This is around ten times more than it spent in 1948. However, costs have risen greatly (particularly the costs of new drugs and treatments), as well as demand. The UK's population is increasing and people are living longer.
- The NHS today is facing various problems. This includes long waiting times, staff shortages, and not enough hospital beds.

Key terms — Make sure you can write a definition for these key terms: Booth, absolute poverty, Rowntree, Boer War, council housing, slum housing, social services, Welfare State

Retrieval

Learn the answers to the questions below, then cover the answers column with a piece of paper and write down as many as you can. Check and repeat.

Questions / Answers

1. What was the title of Charles Booth's 1889 report? — *Life and Labour of the People in London*
2. In which city did Seebohm Rowntree investigate poverty in 1900? — York
3. Why did the government launch the inquiry that led to the Fitzroy Report? — Because around 40 per cent of the men who volunteered to fight in the Boer War were too unfit to be soldiers
4. Which party won the general election in 1906? — The Liberal Party
5. What social reform did the government introduce in 1906 to improve the health of children? — The School Meals Act, which introduced free school meals for children living in poverty
6. What did the government ban in 1909? — The building of back-to-back housing
7. What helped to address the housing shortages after the wars? — Local councils starting building council housing for poorer families
8. What are the 'five giants' named in the Beveridge Report? — Disease, idleness, ignorance, want, and squalor (poor living conditions)
9. How many copies of the Beveridge Report were sold in its first month of publication? — Over 100,000
10. In which year was the NHS introduced? — 1948
11. By how much did life expectancy increase between 1948 and 2019? — By an average of 13 years
12. What did the '5 A Day' campaign encourage people to do? — Eat more fruit and vegetables
13. In 1951, what did the NHS introduce charges for? — Prescriptions, eye care, and dental care

Previous questions

Use the questions below to check your knowledge from previous chapters.

Questions / Answers

1. Why did the Industrial Revolution lead to overcrowding in towns and cities? — Because people left the countryside to take jobs in the new factories that were being built in urban areas across Britain
2. Why were pharmaceutical businesses able to scale up at the end of the nineteenth century? — Because of advances in science and technology, such as the invention of a tablet-making machine in 1843 and a gelatine pill capsule in 1875
3. What does keyhole surgery involve? — Tiny cameras and instruments are inserted into the body through small cuts in the skin

9 Modern public health

Practice

Exam-style questions

Study **Source A**.

Source A: One of a series of posters produced by the NHS in 2022. The poster was part of the 'Better health: let's do this' campaign, which aimed to encourage people to exercise more.

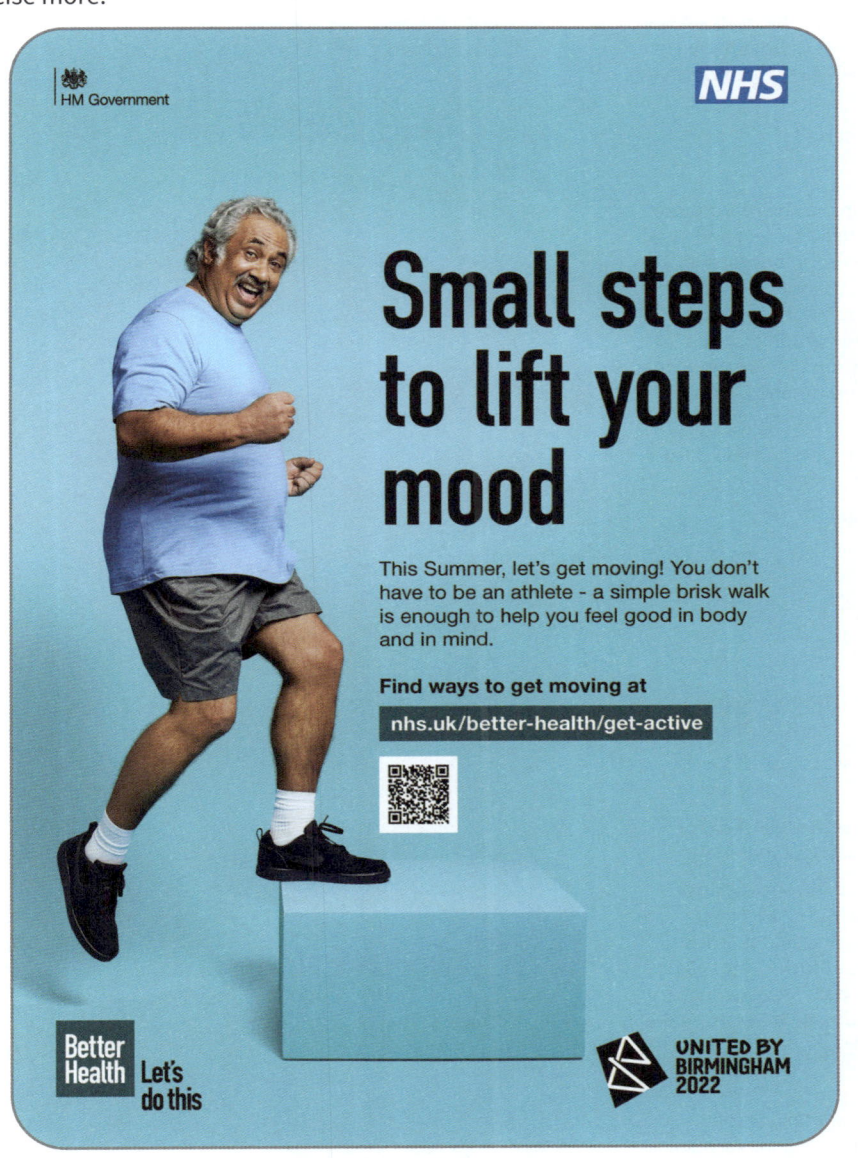

1. How useful is **Source A** to an historian studying the National Health Service? Explain your answer using **Source A** and your contextual knowledge. **(8)**

2. Explain the significance of the work of social reformers to public health. **(8)**

3. Explain **two ways** in which public health reforms in the nineteenth century and public health reforms in the twentieth century were similar. **(8)**

4. Has communication been the main factor in the development of public health in Britain? Explain your answer with reference to the role of communication and other factors. Use a range of examples from across your study of Health and the people: c1000 to the present day. **(16)**

> **EXAM TIP**
>
> Social reformers are people who try to improve society, particularly for those living in poverty, such as Chadwick, Booth, and Rowntree. Consider the ways in which social reformers over the course of history have encouraged the government to improve public health.

OXFORD
UNIVERSITY PRESS

Great Clarendon Street, Oxford, OX2 6DP, United Kingdom

Oxford University Press is a department of the University of Oxford. It furthers the University's objective of excellence in research, scholarship, and education by publishing worldwide. Oxford is a registered trade mark of Oxford University Press in the UK and in certain other countries.

© Oxford University Press 2024

Written by Harriet Power

Series Editor: Aaron Wilkes

The publisher would like to thank Aaron Wilkes for his work on the updated edition of Oxford AQA GCSE History (9–1): Britain: Health and the People c1000–Present Day (978-138-202310-8) on which this revision guide is based.

The moral rights of the author have been asserted

First published in 2024

All rights reserved. No part of this publication may be reproduced, stored in a retrieval system, or transmitted, used for text and data mining, or used for training artificial intelligence, in any form or by any means, without the prior permission in writing of Oxford University Press, or as expressly permitted by law, by licence or under terms agreed with the appropriate reprographics rights organization. Enquiries concerning reproduction outside the scope of the above should be sent to the Rights Department, Oxford University Press, at the address above.

You must not circulate this work in any other form and you must impose this same condition on any acquirer

British Library Cataloguing in Publication Data

Data available

978-1-382-05367-9

978-1-382-05368-6 (ebook)

10 9 8 7 6 5 4 3

The manufacturing process conforms to the environmental regulations of the country of origin.

Printed in the UK by Bell and Bain Ltd, Glasgow

Acknowledgements
The publisher and authors would like to thank the following for permission to use photographs and other copyright material:

Photos: p7: GRANGER - Historical Picture Archive / Alamy Stock Photo; **p11:** Well/BOT / Alamy Stock Photo; **p15:** The History Emporium / Alamy Stock Photo; **p21:** The Trustees of the British Museum; **p27:** Science History Images / Alamy Stock Photo; **p31:** Science History Images / Alamy Stock Photo; **p35:** Steve Greenberg; **p39:** Science Photo Library / Alamy Stock Photo; **p43:** Better Health / Every Mind Matters / Crown copyright.

Artwork by Q2A Media.

Every effort has been made to contact copyright holders of material reproduced in this book. Any omissions will be rectified in subsequent printings if notice is given to the publisher.

Links to third party websites are provided by Oxford in good faith and for information only. Oxford disclaims any responsibility for the materials contained in any third party website referenced in this work.

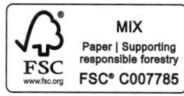

The manufacturer's authorised representative in the EU for product safety is Oxford University Press España S.A. of El Parque Empresarial San Fernando de Henares, Avenida de Castilla, 2 – 28830 Madrid (www.oup.es/en or product.safety@oup.com). OUP España S.A. also acts as importer into Spain of products made by the manufacturer.